100 Ideas for Primary Teachers:

Sensory Processing Differences

Other titles in the 100 Ideas for Primary Teachers series:

100 Ideas for Primary Teachers:

Sensory Processing Differences

Kim Griffin

BLOOMSBURY EDUCATION

LONDON OXFORD NEW YORK NEW DELHI SYDNEY

BLOOMSBURY EDUCATION

Bloomsbury Publishing Plc

50 Bedford Square, London, WC1B 3DP, UK

29 Earlsfort Terrace, Dublin 2, Ireland

BLOOMSBURY, BLOOMSBURY EDUCATION and the Diana logo are
trademarks of Bloomsbury Publishing Plc

First published in Great Britain, 2021 by Bloomsbury Publishing Plc

Bloomsbury Publishing Plc does not have any control over, or responsibility
for, any third-party websites referred to or in this book. All internet addresses
given in this book were correct at the time of going to press. The author and
publisher regret any inconvenience caused if addresses have changed or sites
have ceased to exist, but can accept no responsibility for any such changes

A catalogue record for this book is available from the British Library

ISBN: PB: 978-1-4729-8694-8; ePDF: 978-1-4729-8693-1;
ePub: 978-1-4729-8691-7

2 4 6 8 10 9 7 5 3 1

Typeset by Newgen KnowledgeWorks Pvt. Ltd., Chennai, India
Printed and bound in the UK by CPI Group Ltd, CR0 4YY

To find out more about our authors and books visit www.bloomsbury.com
and sign up for our newsletters.

Contents

Acknowledgements

I would like to firstly thank Susan O'Connor, author of *100 Ideas for Early Years Practitioners: Supporting Children with SEND*, for introducing me to the 100 Ideas series. When she asked me to review her book, I had no idea this would be catalyst for me to also be joining the 100 Ideas series. She has always been very generous with her time and sharing of her publication experiences.

Secondly, I would like to thank the publishing team at Bloomsbury. I would like to express special thanks to Hannah Marston for her enthusiasm and guidance with the book right from our first email.

Thanks to Sue Allen for her thoughts on the initial manuscript and to Karen Leigh Anderson for her guidance and wisdom over the past two years.

Last, but definitely not least, the biggest thanks goes out to all of the amazing therapists I have had the opportunity to learn from throughout my career and the hundreds of children, parents and teachers who have allowed me to use this learning and taught me many things along the way.

Introduction

As usual, I am writing this introduction at the end. The book is in its final draft, the 100 ideas are written. And I am very excited to be sharing it with you.

Sensory processing is a more widely recognised concept nowadays. Research reports that somewhere between one in 20 and one in 6.25 children may experience sensory processing difficulties (Crasta et al., 2020). This means that in a classroom of 30 children, between two and five pupils may process sensory information differently.

These pupils are already sitting in your classroom. This book offers information and strategies you can use to support them. The ideas will likely be helpful for pupils who have a diagnosis of autism, developmental coordination disorder or attention deficit hyperactivity disorder (ADHD), as these pupils often experience sensory differences. They can also support pupils without a formal diagnosis who you think might have sensory needs.

The book has been written for readers at all stages of their journey in learning about sensory processing. For teachers who are new to sensory processing, you may want to spend more time in Parts 1 and 2 to familiarise yourself with the terms. Teachers with some experience supporting sensory needs may wish to go straight to the later parts of the book where specific ideas are covered.

I would recommend that all readers review Part 3. Here, I cover the reasons why you will be using sensory supports. Part 3 will help you to set targets and monitor outcomes. This is an important step, which should not be forgotten.

A note on terminology

Throughout the book, I will use the term sensory processing. I have chosen to use this term because it is a more widely known term. However, I wish to make the reader aware of two important points. Firstly, sensory processing disorder is not recognised as a formal stand-alone diagnosis. Sensory differences, like hypo- or hyper-responsivity, are recognised within the autism diagnostic criteria. However, it is still not a formally recognised condition.

Secondly, we would not be using the term sensory processing without the work of Dr A. Jean Ayres. Dr Ayres is the founder of sensory integration theory. She spent the best part of her working life developing her theory and the Ayres Sensory Integration® treatment approach. Without her work, subsequent authors would not have coined the term sensory processing.

These days the terms sensory processing and sensory integration are often used interchangeably. I would like to take this opportunity to inform the reader that there are differences within the two models. Whilst some definitions are given throughout the book, explaining the differences in these two models fully is outside of the scope of this book. It is also not necessary for readers to understand these models in depth to use the strategies offered in this book. However, it is helpful for the reader to know that researchers within the field have taken diverged paths. And in the future, with the publication of new research, the terminology and models may change again.

Sensory preferences

We all have different sensory preferences. Some people love the smell of coffee, others don't. Some of us like going on rollercoasters, the rest of us like to keep our feet firmly planted on the ground. For individuals with sensory processing differences, their interpretation of sensation is more than just a preference. Sometimes sensations can be painful, sometimes they are distracting. In some cases the sensation might trigger a fight, flight or freeze response. For others, the sensation may not even register. There is no right or wrong, there is just the experience for that individual.

In the classroom, typically a resulting behaviour will be observed. For example, the sensation of touch might trigger a child to hit their peer; a loud sound might result in the child running away; or a need for movement might result in the child rocking in their chair.

Sometimes, behaviour will be behaviour. Sometimes it might be that the child is hungry, tired or sick. However, sometimes the behaviour you are seeing is an outward expression of a sensory need.

Your challenge

The challenge I set you is to start applying your sensory goggles. Use the introductory information in Parts 1 and 2 of this book to better understand the senses. Add the question 'Could it be sensory?' into your observations. Keep your sensory goggles on.

Use the strategies in the later parts of the book to test your assumptions. If it is a sensory issue, they should help. Sometimes they are not only helpful for the pupil with the sensory needs, but they can also be a useful support for the whole class.

Good luck on your sensory journey.

How to use this book

This book includes quick, easy and practical ideas for you to dip in and out of to help you support pupils with sensory processing differences.

Each idea includes:

- a catchy title, easy to refer to and share with your colleagues
- an interesting quote linked to the idea
- a summary of the idea in bold, making it easy to flick through the book and identify an idea you want to use at a glance
- a step-by-step guide to implementing the idea.

Each idea also includes one or more of the following:

Teaching tip

Practical tips and advice for how and how not to run the activity or put the idea into practice.

Taking it further

Ideas and advice for how to extend the idea or develop it further.

Bonus idea ★

There are 61 bonus ideas in this book that are extra-exciting, extra-original and extra-interesting.

Share how you use these ideas and find out what other practitioners have done using **#100ideas**.

Sensory
foundations

Part 1

Sensory input

'When I started considering it, I was surprised at how many sensory messages a pupil receives every day when they are sitting in my classroom.'

Sensory input refers to any information that the brain receives from the senses. The brain constantly receives sensory inputs from the body and the environment. These include messages received from the important, but lesser known, proprioceptive and vestibular senses.

Sensory inputs ooze from every part of your classroom. There are wall displays, there are the sounds of pupils and adults, there are different materials to feel and work with and there is the constant movement of books, pens and people. In addition to this, each pupil is processing the sensory inputs from their own body (Idea 7). Sensory inputs are essential for learning, but can also be a source of distraction and for some a barrier to success.

When you have a moment, sit in your classroom and pay attention to every sensory input that occurs. What can you see, hear, touch and smell? As you move through a typical day, really consider how your senses are helping, or not helping, you to be successful. Your touch sense helps every time you use the smart board. Your vestibular sense (Idea 6) helps you to keep your balance when you sit up and move about. Your proprioceptive sense (Idea 5) helps you to know how much pressure to use when you write. You're constantly looking at and listening to your pupils.

This book explores different ways your pupils may process sensory inputs occurring in your classroom and within their own bodies. Throughout the book, you must always start by thinking about sensory inputs, because these are the key to selecting the right support.

Sight

'It is remarkable how much of the day-to-day learning in a classroom requires the pupil to visually attend and to switch their visual attention between activities.'

The sense of sight, or visual sense, is essential for learning in most classrooms. It allows pupils to read the board and to look at teacher demonstrations. It helps with communication. In addition, it's important for writing, cutting and success in the playground.

The sensory input received by the vision sense is light. There are special receptors at the back of the eye, called cones and rods, which respond to light. They receive information about the colours, movement and shape of objects. This sensory input is then processed by the brain. Standard vision assessments test visual acuity. This relates to the clearness of the image the brain receives and it can be corrected with glasses. However, it is only part of the story.

Some pupils might have challenges with visual discrimination or vision perception. This relates to how the pupil's brain interprets what they are seeing. Examples include discriminating between letters (e.g. 'b' from 'd') and symbols (e.g. '+' from 'x'). These pupils will need more support to develop their visual perception. Other pupils might also have difficulty paying adequate visual attention or looking in the right place! For example, you may start demonstrating something with your hands, but they are still looking at the board. So, they miss important information. These pupils benefit from additional verbal cues of exactly where they need to be looking. Finally, some pupils have difficulty ignoring irrelevant visual information (e.g. the gardener outside). These pupils typically need visual distractions in the environment to be reduced (Idea 40).

Teaching tip

Peripheral (or side) vision can be used to gain attention more quickly. Try bringing the information in from the left or right side of the pupil's face, rather than presenting it directly in front of them.

Taking it further

Puzzles, matching worksheets, visual games and books like *Where's Wally?* can sometimes help those who have difficulties in visual perception or discrimination, while privacy screens can be useful for those who are easily visually distracted.

Hearing

'It feels like I am speaking all day long when I am in class. This means my pupils must be doing a lot of listening.'

The sense of hearing, or auditory sense, is also crucial for learning in most classrooms. Pupils need to listen to what their teacher is saying. They need to listen to videos, music and other instructions. They are also listening to their peers. Adequate listening skills are vital for schooling success.

As you will likely know, the receptor for hearing is the cochlear. This is part of the inner ear and it processes the sound waves that are received from the environment. The speed of the sound wave determines the frequency of the sound. The sound waves enter the ear, travel to the ear drum and make it vibrate. The brain then interprets these vibrations as sounds.

The auditory sense helps to orientate us to our environment. Some pupils find locating and identifying sounds more challenging. Or, they might speak too loudly as they don't discriminate volume of sound very well. Some pupils have difficulty paying attention to the right noises, e.g. the teacher talking. They may become distracted by irrelevant sounds. Others might be slower to register that sounds have occurred. Sound sensitivity can also occur (Idea 13) and this might lead to overload (Idea 32). In all cases, the pupil misses out on learning.

It can be helpful to identify whether the pupil is sensitive to sounds or less aware of them. If a pupil is less aware, greater variety, volume and variance in pitch may help. Some pupils may also benefit from a sound cue (e.g. a bell or a clap) to draw their attention. Listening for the direction of sounds with their eyes closed can also be a way to help pupils to identify direction of sounds.

Touch

'I was amazed to learn that the skin is the largest organ in the human body!'

Whilst it might not be the most obvious sense to help with learning, the touch sense is just as important as hearing and vision. The touch sense also supports coordination. In order to hold a pencil, cut with scissors and do up their buttons, a pupil must have a well-developed sense of touch.

An important thing to understand about the touch sense is that it receives sensory inputs from the skin. Anything that touches the skin will activate the touch receptors. In addition, the skin also receives information about pain, temperature, touch pressure and vibration.

Different parts of the body have a different number of receptors, the cells in the body that receive the sensory information. The hands, face and mouth have more receptors than the face and back. This explains why some parts of the skin are more sensitive than others. Touch receptors in the mouth help with chewing, swallowing food and talking.

The touch sense is very important for a number of reasons. Firstly, like the other senses, it plays a protective role. Secondly, it helps with soothing and calming. For example, a baby will usually stop crying when it is held. Finally, the touch sense is essential for pupils to be able to use their hands and to use tools. This might be a pencil or scissors or cutlery.

Pupils who are slower to process touch sensory inputs are often clumsier than their peers. Dr A. Jean Ayres, who developed the theory of sensory integration, found a link between dyspraxia (Idea 10) and the touch sense. Some individuals are more sensitive to touch than others. This is called tactile defensiveness (see Idea 14).

Taking it further

If you want to understand more about the protective and discriminative touch sense, they are explored in more detail in the GriffinOT online introduction to sensory processing. See: www.GriffinOT.com/100ideas.

Proprioception

'I was always confused as to why she used too much pressure, broke things and petted the dog with so much force. Once I understood proprioception it all made sense!'

Proprioception is essential to know where the body parts are in space. It is commonly referred to as body awareness and often called the 'hidden sixth sense'.

The proprioceptive sense lets the brain know where the limbs are in space and how they are moving. For example, when you walk, you don't need to look at where your feet are. Your proprioceptive sense helps your brain to 'feel' your legs and feet.

The receptors for the proprioceptive sense are in the muscles and joints of the body and limbs. This is what separates it from the touch sense, which receives sensory inputs from the skin. The proprioceptive sense receives information about muscle stretch, joint loading and joint compression, which tells the brain about the position of the joint and the amount of force or pressure being used. The proprioceptors are responsible for squeezing, pushing and pulling with the right amount of force for the task.

Pupils with proprioceptive difficulties may use too much or too little force or pressure. They might hold their pencil really loosely and press really lightly or press so hard the pencil lead breaks. In the playground, they may struggle to control the amount of force they use when they kick or throw a ball. Often pupils with reduced proprioceptive awareness will move into others' space, walk into peers or stretch across them without noticing. When walking, they might touch the wall to help them to orientate their bodies. They will likely hug with too much force and go through their glue stick very quickly.

Vestibular

'I never knew that the balance sense also helped with coordination, control of eye movements and understanding speed of movement, and that it supported attention.'

The vestibular sense is often called our movement or balance sense. Like proprioception, it is a lesser-known sense. It is working tirelessly in the background to help with balance, coordination, attention, stillness and movement. It also helps with emotional regulation.

The receptors for this sense sit in the middle ear in a part called the vestibule. This is where the vestibular system gets its name. This organ processes information about head movement. It lets the brain know how fast the head is moving, which direction it is going and how high it is off the ground. Adequate processing of this information is required for balance and movement. Functionally, it supports postural control and coordination.

In addition to supporting balance, the vestibular system helps to control visual attention and eye movements and to keep our gaze steady. This includes the ability to scan when reading and also to shift focus between the board, the teacher and work on the pupil's desk during lessons. It also helps to maintain alertness and attention.

When sitting in the classroom, a pupil is constantly relying on their vestibular sense. The vestibular sense helps them to sit upright and to have enough endurance to stay seated for an entire lesson. Some pupils might move about and rock on their chair when this sense isn't working well (Idea 7).

Teaching tip

Individuals who have problems processing vestibular information often rely on vision to support their balance. This means that they struggle with their balance more when they have to then use their eyes to look at something else, like a ball. So they are much more likely to fall over or trip or be quite uncoordinated in PE.

Taking it further

Too much vestibular sensory input can make a pupil feel sick. Everyone has different thresholds. There are those who love to be on the rides and to spin, and others who hate it, and this is because everyone has different thresholds for vestibular sensory input.

Interoception

'It's all about what is going on inside. It's strange that we don't immediately think about the huge impact this has on behaviour and self-regulation. Sometimes we look for complex reasons, but actually it may be a simple answer.'

Interoception refers to the sensory input that the brain receives internally from the body. The information comes from the organs and internal receptors. It includes sensations regarding hunger, needing the toilet, tiredness, sickness and internal pain such as a stomach ache or headache. It is very important as it facilitates the awareness and regulation of one's internal state.

Teaching tip

If there is a significant change in a pupil's behaviour in a short space of time, it is useful to consider their internal sensations. They may be getting sick, or may be tired, or could have a toothache. Sometimes, it might be an internal, rather than external, sensation.

The receptors for interoception are in the internal organs, nerves and pain receptors. Because this sensory feedback is received internally from the body, it is much harder for educators to see or notice and it can sometimes be overlooked.

If pupils are not processing this internal information very well, or at all, they may not recognise when they are hungry or if they need to go to the toilet – or they may recognise too late and then it's a rush to get there! They may be in discomfort or pain but not identify that this is occurring. A pupil might not recognise that they are too hot; therefore they won't take their jumper off and they will be uncomfortable.

Like all of the senses, awareness or lack of awareness of the interoceptive sense can have a big impact on attention and focus, and subsequent ability to participate and engage. If pupils are not processing this internal information accurately, they may appear to have an emotional reaction without any warning. This is especially important to consider for pupils who are non-verbal or who have reduced communication as they have even less capacity to explain what is going on.

Sensory processing or sensory integration

'Sensory integration is the organisation of the senses for use.' Dr A. Jean Ayres (2005, p. 5)

Sensory processing or sensory integration relates to the way the brain interprets the sensory input, or messages, that it receives.

The term 'sensory integration' (SI) was first used by occupational therapist Dr A. Jean Ayres in 1950. After noticing that the pupils she was working with were processing sensory information differently, Dr Ayres developed her treatment approach. This pupil-led approach helps pupils' brains to better understand and organise, or integrate, sensory inputs. In the 2000s, there was a shift to using the term 'sensory processing disorder' (SPD). This term was initially published by Dr Lucy Miller, another occupational therapist. The terms sensory processing and sensory integration are now sometimes used interchangeably. However, theoretically they are represented by different models.

If a pupil is not processing sensory information adequately, you may notice sensitivity to noises or touch, poor body awareness, difficulty in planning and organising new activities/movements, inattention and slower to respond to information, reduced endurance or poor postural control.

SPD is not a formally recognised diagnosis. Sensory hypo- and hyper-responsivity are recognised in the autism diagnostic criteria. Dyspraxia is recognised under developmental coordination disorder (DCD). However, currently there is insufficient evidence to support sensory processing as a standalone diagnosis. SI difficulties are associated with a number of diagnoses but can also be seen independently.

Teaching tip

If you do have concerns about a pupil, speak with your SENDCo. You can also make a referral to an occupational therapist (Idea 29) or other professionals (Idea 30) for further advice.

Taking it further

This video describes sensory processing from a pupil's perspective: www.youtube.com/watch?v=D1G5ssZlVUw.

Bonus idea ★

If the reader wanted to understand the models in further depth, please see the book recommendations in the Further reading section.

Sensory modulation

'There are two pupils in my class who are polar opposites. One overreacts to everything. She can't focus with noise and will flinch if anyone accidently brushes past her. The other is just so slow to respond to everything, it's like watching a slow motion film.'

Sensory modulation is the ability to match your responses and behaviour to the environment, activity and/or situation. It is the brain's ability to process the sensory inputs, or messages, from the body and produce a response that is in proportion to the input. It needs to match the level of intensity and the environment.

Teaching tip

It is important to remember that pupils can have different responses with different senses. They might be more sensitive to touch but slower to respond to proprioceptive sensory input. It is rare that there is a neat pattern of sensitive, seeking or slower across all senses. Remember, responses will fluctuate depending on overall arousal (Idea 21).

Taking it further

The book *Sensational Kids* by Dr Lucy Jane Miller explores the concepts in much further depth.

In the literature, sensory modulation differences are broken into two, three or four 'subtypes' depending on the author. All authors agree that there is a continuum of responses from low to highly reactive. They just present their models slightly differently. In this book we will stick with three subtypes: sensitive, slower and seeking.

Sensitive (over-responsive)

Pupils who are sensitive have lower thresholds for sensory inputs than others. This means that they can be quickly overloaded (Idea 32) by sensory information. There might be sensitivities to sound (Idea 13), touch (Idea 14) or movement (Idea 15) and also food fussiness (Idea 39).

For them, sensory inputs can also trigger a fight, flight or freeze response. Externally, you may observe these pupils hitting out, running away, engaging in avoidance or shutting down (Idea 32). Internally, what is occurring is that the pupils' brains are being overwhelmed by the sensory inputs they are receiving.

If have already read Idea 1, you should have some appreciation of the sheer number of sensory inputs occurring in your classroom. Pupils who are sensitive will notice even more sensory inputs than you! If they are verbal, you can ask them what they notice. One boy I worked with could identify blue and white chalk by smell. If they are non-verbal, it's your job to identify what sensory inputs might be triggers. The starting point for individuals who are sensitive is to help to decrease their arousal (Idea 24).

Slower (under-responsive)

Pupils who are slower to respond can often be missed. This is because they are usually quiet and blend into the background easily and are missing out on learning opportunities. It's important that you look out for them! These pupils will take more time to notice sensory inputs. Their response may be slower. They may also have poor posture (Idea 17 and Idea 56). They often need help to increase their arousal (Idea 26).

Seeking

Sensory seekers are easy to spot. They are the pupils who are rocking on their chairs, or always touching or fiddling with things on their desk. They might use too much force and always be seeking out more push or pull. They are typically the ones that like harder, faster and bigger sensory inputs. Typically, sensory seekers need support to help to organise their systems; this is explored further in Idea 25.

Other considerations

Sometimes, sensory behaviours are not as straight forward as they may appear. A pupil might be 'seeking' sensory inputs from one sense in an effort to compensate for another. For example, they might appear to be seeking out extra auditory input because they are making noises. However, they are actually making their own noise to drown out other sounds in the classroom. Or they might be touching everything to compensate for slower responses from their proprioceptive sense (Idea 5).

Pupils can have different reactivity or responses with different senses. Responses can fluctuate with anxiety, tiredness and hunger. They will also change as the pupil matures.

Bonus idea

An occupational therapist (Idea 29) can help with identifying sensory input triggers for those who are sensitive. They can also help to identify the important distinction between seeking sensory inputs and trying to compensate for other sensory processing differences.

Dyspraxia

'Once I understood about planning and ideation, dyspraxia made a lot more sense.'

Dyspraxia is a term used to describe the difficulty pupils and adults have when they struggle to plan and organise their movements. It is sometimes used interchangeably with the term developmental coordination disorder (DCD). This is because dyspraxia itself isn't a formally recognised medical diagnosis, whereas DCD is.

Teaching tip

Teaching pupils to ask for help when they don't understand is a really helpful strategy.

Despite frequent misuse of the term, dyspraxia is much more than just a little clumsiness. It is expected that those with dyspraxia would have difficulties with thinking of and organising their ideas rather than just doing them. In fact, there are three components of dyspraxia.

1. **Ideation**. Ideation means coming up with an idea or having the idea of what to do. For example, if you have a box of LEGO®, you need to think of what you want to build.
2. **Planning**. Planning is the ability to figure out how to do the idea, including organising the steps and movements of an activity. To build a house with LEGO®, you need to decide where and in which order to put the bricks.
3. **Doing**. Doing is the part where your body moves. With LEGO®, this includes pressing the bricks together and using the right amount of pressure.

Taking it further

Often, pupils with dyspraxia don't generalise learning from one task to another. This means you can't assume they will understand an activity because it's similar to one they did previously. Sometimes, they need instructions from the beginning each time.

Pupils may have difficulty with ideation, planning or both, and you need to consider which of these they are finding challenging. Idea 50 discusses ideation and Ideas 51 and 52 give strategies for planning.

Pupils experience the most difficulty when they are learning a new task, especially complex tasks so they will need more support, time and practice initially to learn something new.

How differences present

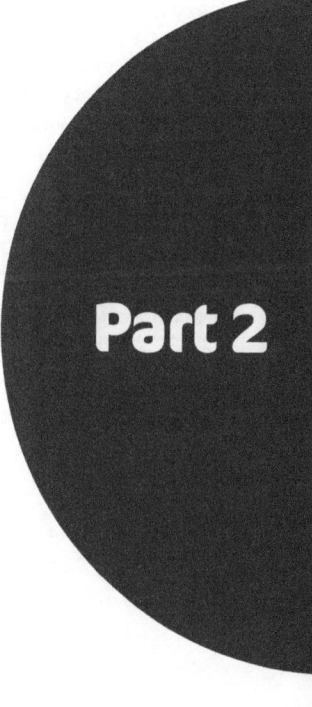

Part 2

Sensory or behaviour?

'Every pupil you meet who experiences sensory differences will present differently. There is no exact pattern or processing style. You will need to get to know the individual.'

It is very common for sensory differences to be seen as behaviour externally. Easily observable behaviours could include avoidance, anger or distress. However, some individuals internalise their behaviour, so they may become quiet or disengage. It's important to consider both ways of responding.

Teaching tip

Keeping a home–school diary to record any changes at home can also help with spotting patterns. Sometimes it might be a change at home that is causing the behaviour change at school, e.g. if the family has visitors staying.

Sensory differences may present as a modulation difficulty (Idea 9), dyspraxia (Idea 10), poor balance (Idea 17) or a combination of these. Modulation difficulties may result in things like sound sensitivity, avoidance of messy play, seeking of additional movement or food fussiness. Dyspraxia and poor balance typically lead to poor coordination and challenges with motor skills and planning. The first step in identifying sensory behaviours is being aware of them. Parts 2 and 3 of this book outline many of the common behaviours that could indicate there is difficulty processing sensory inputs. If you are familiar with these, you will be able to identify sensory behaviours more readily. The next step is to determine whether the behaviour has an observable sensory origin. Not everything will be sensory. Sometimes, there are communication difficulties or the behaviour is driven by another need such as pain, attachment issues or attention. Sometimes, pupils will just be pushing the boundary. The ABC and STAR models can help with observation, both of which give a clear structure for considering behaviours.

ABC

Antecedent: What happened before the behaviour occurred? Consider the

Bonus idea ★

For further advice on identifying whether the behaviour is due to sensory processing differences, you could also refer to an occupational therapist (Idea 29).

environment, task and people in the space as well. Make sure you consider the adult's actions as well as the pupil's.

Behaviour: What was the observable behaviour? Consider exactly what the behaviour looked like and whether any particular people (adults or pupils) were involved.

Consequence: What occurred afterwards? Consider both the pupil and adult's actions. Sometimes, we inadvertently promote behaviour due to the consequence we give the pupil. For example, pupils who have sensitivities may prefer to go and sit outside the headteacher's office rather than go to PE, so cause a problem in order to go to the quiet space rather than be in a loud and busy one. What the adult perceives as a consequence, the pupil perceives as a reward.

STAR

The STAR model is very similar but breaks the observations down under different headings.

Setting: Where the behaviour happened. Consider the space, people and task.

Trigger: What triggered or led to the behaviour? Consider both sensory inputs and interactions with others.

Action: What behaviour occurred? What did the pupil do?

Result: What was the consequence? This includes how others reacted. Sometimes, individuals with poor communication skills will repeat behaviours in order to receive a response or reaction. They may be trying to interact with their peers, but as they don't have language skills they might hit out so their peer pays attention to them.

Keep a record

The easiest way to remember behaviours and triggers is to keep a record. The record can help you to identify whether there are any patterns to the antecedent/trigger or consequence/result, so you know what to change.

Taking it further

It is common for sensory behaviours, especially for children with autism, to exacerbate at times of illness. Often, this occurs a couple of days before the pupil is obviously unwell so make sure you include illness in your record, as sometimes it's the trigger.

Teaching tip

Choose a record keeping format that best suits your workplace and keep a record of events. It's useful to note down additional things like tiredness, illness, holidays and changes in routine as these may have an impact.

Flight, fight, freeze

'He would always run off if there was a siren. I realised much later that it was his fight-flight-freeze response rather than him just having no awareness.'

The 'fight-flight-freeze response' is an automatic response the brain makes in order to keep the body safe. It is the reflex that moves your hand away if you touch something hot or if you step on a thorn. Some pupils may have this response to certain sensory inputs. The response is reflexive.

The first thing to remember when helping pupils who experience a fight-flight-freeze response is that they do not have much control over their response. Their response is automatic. Understanding this can help your own frustration level and also help you to plan how to help the pupil.

Pre-warning where possible can help to reduce the pupil's reaction. This is not always going to be possible but it's a big help when you can. This is because it prepares the pupil's brain so the sensory input won't be a surprise, as they are expecting it.

If it is a sensory input that the pupil could have control over, letting them play with it can be helpful. For example, if it was a musical instrument, a bell or a light, they could use it themselves first. Please do not just expose the pupil to the sensory input with the expectation that this will decrease their response. This can actually make their response worse.

Finally, it's important to remember that because this is a reflexive reaction, the pupil will have much less control over it. A behavioural approach expecting them to inhibit their response will likely be unsuccessful.

Hearing sensitivity

'It was like he had supersonic hearing. Everything was a distraction, even the whir of the projector in the room.'

Hearing or auditory sensitivity is a very commonly reported sensory processing difference. It is frequently reported by those with autism.

Sensitivity to sounds is an example of poor sensory modulation (Idea 9). The pupil's brain is paying more attention to the sounds and has more difficulty filtering out background noise in the environment. Often they can be quickly overwhelmed by sound. Here are some specific strategies you can use to help:

- Where possible, reduce the noise in the classroom.
- Position the pupil away from other pupils who might make noise.
- Prepare pupils for noise that might occur, e.g. if there will be music.
- Warn them that you are going to make a loud sound before you make it.
- Let them have control over new sounds, e.g. musical instruments, whistles or bells.
- Ear defenders or ear plugs can sometimes help (Idea 77). For pupils with larger heads, gardening headphones are a useful option.
- Noise-cancelling headphones can be used without music playing.
- Music therapies, e.g. Tomatis ®, The Listening Programme or Therapeutic Listening, are offered by some professionals (e.g. OTs).

Finally, it is very important to remember that the impact of noise can be cumulative. If you know the pupil is sensitive to sounds, make sure you give them quiet breaks between noisier activities. Assembly, music lessons, PE halls and lunch are often much louder times of the day, so try not to have them back to back.

Teaching tip

Sometimes pupils who are sensitive to sounds make their own noises to cover up sounds in the environment. Monitor when the sounds occur and this might help to give you a clue whether they are sensitive to or seeking more noise.

Taking it further

Watch this video 'Autism and sound sensitivity' by The National Autistic Society: www.youtube.com/watch?v=ycCN3qTYVyo.

Bonus idea ★

You could try some heavy work activities (Idea 59) prior to and after being in a noisy environment, which will help to calm the individual's nervous system.

Touch sensitivity

'He always avoids having messy hands and won't play with things like sand.'

Touch sensitivity is a commonly reported sensory processing difference. The sensitivity is usually to lighter touch and tickle sensations. It can lead to food fussiness (Idea 39), avoidance of messy play and difficulties with the feeling of clothing, shoes, hair cutting, hair brushing and tooth brushing.

When there is touch sensitivity, you must be mindful that certain touch sensations may register as painful for the pupil. Others may cause a fight-flight-freeze response (Idea 12) so the pupil is not wholly in control of their behavioural responses. This means that you will likely have more success supporting the pupil with sensory strategies rather than a behavioural approach. Here are some specific strategies you can use to help:

- Always tell the pupil before going to touch them that you are going to touch them and where, e.g. 'Sarah I'm just going to touch your hand to help you hold the scissors correctly.'
- Position the pupil on the edges of groups or the back of the line so that there are fewer chances for accidental touch.
- Use a firmer touch pressure (Idea 44).
- Increase opportunities for the pupil to engage in messy play and to explore different textures (Idea 43).
- Use heavy work activities (Idea 59) before and after a touch activity the pupil finds difficult.

The final section of this book includes additional ideas for self-care tasks like hair brushing and dressing, which individuals with touch sensitivity can sometimes find a challenge.

Teaching tip

Because these pupils can experience accidental touch as painful or more forceful than it was intended, they may need support to understand when another pupil has accidently touched them that it was an accident. This can be especially true in sports as they may perceive another pupil as being very rough even if they were just playing the game as expected.

Taking it further

GriffinOT's free online introduction to sensory processing explores the touch sense in further depth, explaining why sensitivity may occur. See www.GriffinOT.com/100ideas.

Movement sensitivity

'She always avoids the playground equipment; I have never seen a pupil so fearful of a swing.'

Movement sensitivity can occur when a pupil experiences sensitivity to vestibular input (Idea 6).

Often movement sensitivity results in an avoidance of equipment that moves, like swings and slides. Some pupils cannot manage when their feet come off the ground so may avoid things like climbing frames, scooters and bicycles. They may also dislike being lifted up into the air and heights.

The first tip here is to let the pupil be in charge of the movement. Never force them into movement that they are not comfortable with. This might trigger a fight-fight-freeze response (Idea 12). Giving them control will make them feel safer. It will also build trust.

You can SLOWLY encourage them to explore a bit further each time, but always let them have control and respect their choices. If you are helping to make the movement, ALWAYS STOP when they ask to or after the number you have said you would. This builds trust and also confidence.

Sitting on a large exercise or yoga ball for short periods can help to increase tolerance to movement. Make sure the pupil can firmly place their feet on the ground. You may need to secure the ball initially so it doesn't move. The ball will be more stable if it is slightly deflated. Let the pupil slowly increase the amount of time they can sit on it. They can also march, rock side to side, bounce and try to balance on one foot when they are more comfortable.

Teaching tip

The pupil will feel safer if their feet can touch the ground, so make swings and bicycles lower. For equipment that moves, try to make it more stable or slower initially until the pupil's confidence increases.

Taking it further

Direct sensory integration therapy (Idea 31) can make a real difference for pupils with movement sensitivity; a referral to an occupational therapist should be considered (Idea 29).

Movement seeking

'These pupils are usually the first ones referred to therapists as they stand out in class, because they often rock, move, spin and hop in and out of their chair.'

Contrary to what might be the initial observation, pupils who seek out additional movement are thought to have lower levels of arousal (Idea 21). They are using the movement to help to increase their alertness. Sometimes, they may have poor body awareness (Idea 54) and/or posture (Idea 56). Some pupils with autism might be using movement to stim (Idea 35).

In the classroom, a movement-seeking pupil will likely be the one rocking on their chair, or they might be tapping their pencils or fidgeting with items on their desk. They usually get up to approach the teacher more frequently.

It's useful to check whether the pupil is paying attention when they are moving. Often, the movement helps the pupil's attention. If you expect them to stay still, they have to focus their attention on staying still. Then, they can't focus on their learning.

This is where structured movement opportunities or equipment can be helpful. These are explored in the following ideas:

- marking out a space/boundary (Idea 55)
- keeping lunchtime (Idea 58)
- movement minutes (Idea 60)
- sensory diets (Idea 61)
- sensory circuits (Idea 62)
- structured movement (Idea 63)
- animal walks (Idea 64)
- wobble cushions (Idea 70)
- scooter boards (Idea 78).

Poor balance and coordination

'Her balance was really poor. She really struggled on playground equipment and found it very difficult to learn to use her scooter. And she still can't ride her bike.'

Pupils with slower responses to vestibular and proprioceptive sensory inputs often have poor balance and postural control. This is because their brains respond more slowly to this sensory input, so they are slower to make adjustments with their movements. They can appear clumsy.

Signs of poor postural control include:

- appearing weaker than other pupils their age
- often having a loose grasp on objects and having difficulty turning knobs or handles that require some pressure
- poor balance during PE and other motor activities, like using playground equipment
- difficulty maintaining posture at the table
- poor balance and falling over easily, sometimes even when seated
- difficulty using both hands at the same time
- tiring easily or frequently appearing tired
- having low arousal and reduced attention.

These pupils may need encouragement to join in with physical activity. You may need to provide them with easier activities initially, to help build their confidence and skill. Don't assume they will be able to meet age-related targets. Additional strategies to help are explored in the following ideas:

- low arousal (Idea 49)
- helping posture and core strength (Idea 56)
- bilateral integration (Idea 57)
- wobble cushions (Idea 70)
- therapy balls (Idea 73)
- scooter boards (Idea 78).

Teaching tip

If you have significant concerns about a pupil's balance or coordination, a referral to an occupational therapist or physiotherapist should be considered.

Why are they chewing on everything?

'If it's not his pencil, it's his collar or sleeve. There is just always something in his mouth!'

Chewing is a form of oral sensory seeking. Chewing itself provides a big hit of proprioceptive (Idea 5) sensory input to the brain. This is because the jaw muscle is one of the strongest muscles in the human body. Often individuals who are chewing are trying to regulate, or calm down, their nervous system.

Teaching tip

Oral toys, like instruments or whistles, can help some pupils. Consider increasing the options for chewing and sucking within meals. Chewy food like dried fruit and bagels are great, and you can use a straw for drinks.

Oral sensory seeking is a normal behaviour in babies and infants; it is also known as 'mouthing'. They use sucking to help to calm themselves and self-soothe or self-regulate. Sucking is also an important survival reflex, which is essential for feeding. This behaviour typically stops somewhere between 18 and 24 months. There are five reasons why mouthing continues past this age.

1. The pupil has developmental delays, so cognitively they are still processing information at an 18–24-month-old level. These pupils need more time to develop past this stage and should be provided with sensorimotor play choices. It is also important to ensure that toys given to these pupils are marked 'suitable for under two years old'.

2. The pupil is using the input to self-soothe. Sucking is very calming. It is a strategy that babies use to help self-soothe and regulate. Some pupils continue to use this strategy even when they are older, and it can be a sign that the pupil is upset, tired or overwhelmed. If the behaviour is not impacting functionally on the pupil's engagement and participation, sometimes it can be best to leave it, as stopping it may elicit other unwanted behaviours.

3. The pupil is experiencing sensory overload (Idea 32). In this case, the pupil is using the oral sensory input in an attempt to help to regulate. It's important to consider whether the environment or activity is increasing the pupil's arousal. Look for patterns, e.g. does the pupil chew more during assembly? You can use many of the sensory strategies in this book to help with overall regulation. This might help to decrease the pupil's need to chew or suck. Ideas for chew toys are discussed in Idea 75.

4. In some cases, the pupil may have problems with their teeth. If this is suspected, the pupil should have a check-up with their dentist.

5. The pupil may have a medical condition called 'pica'. Pupils with pica put all things, not just food, into their mouths. They don't distinguish edible and non-edible items. Research has suggested that between four and 26 per cent of people with learning disabilities show pica. Reasons for pica could be medical, dietary, sensory or behavioural and should be investigated further by a medical practitioner.

Taking it further

The West London Mental Health NHS booklet, 'Eating difficulties in children and young people with disabilities' discusses pica on page 23. See: www.wlmht.nhs.uk/wp-content/uploads/2015/01/Eating-difficulties-in-children-with-disabilities.pdf.

Avoidance

'He never joined in with PE and preferred to sit and watch in the playground. It was really hard to get him engaged.'

One response to sensory sensitivities is to avoid situations. This is because the pupil knows the sensation is unpleasant for them, so they avoid putting themselves into the situation. Avoidance is also a strategy used by pupils with dyspraxia and poor balance as it means they will not fail at an activity.

The first step in helping is to identify why the pupil might be avoiding activities, situations or environments. It can be helpful to keep a diary, noting when or what the pupil avoids. Is it a particular subject, a particular piece of playground equipment or a specific play station? It might even be a staff member or specific space. The lunch hall can be overwhelming for some pupils, the PE hall for others.

Take a step back and look for patterns and sensations. Does the pupil always avoid lunch on a specific day? Maybe this is because they don't like the smell of the food, e.g. fish on Fridays. Does the pupil always avoid places that are loud? Do they always try to avoid PE or lunchtime play? Looking at the patterns will help you to determine the underlying reasons. It could be that a sensation is overwhelming. For some pupils, perhaps they don't understand what to do or don't want to be unable to do the activity. Once you understand the triggers, you can start to find solutions.

Bonus idea ★

Allowing the pupil to watch before they join in can sometimes help. This could be watching during the activity but could also be a video of the other pupils completing the activity.

If it's the sensation that is the problem, consider how you can reduce the impact of it. In this book, Part 5 explores ideas to support touch. Part 8 gives extra ideas for regulation and Part 9 considers functional skills. If dyspraxia or postural control is the issue, consider the additional ideas in Part 6.

Not noticing

'He just seems to always be in his own world. His response times take forever.'

Some pupils are much slower to notice sensory inputs. They can appear unengaged or unresponsive. This is because their brain hasn't yet registered or processed the sensations. Typically these pupils benefit from these three supports.

As a first step, it is important to cue their attention. It may be that you call their name and wait until they are looking in the right direction before giving further information. Touching their shoulder to cue them before speaking can help in some cases. Some pupils might cue to a sound or a visual. Each pupil will be different.

Secondly, they typically need more time to respond. This is especially important when giving instructions. Rather than repeating the instruction straight away, wait for longer than you typically would. If they are still processing the information and you give them more, their brain then needs to try to process two pieces of information. This will slow them down further! Even though it might feel like an awkward pause, it's likely the pause is helpful for the pupil.

Finally, these pupils may need a higher intensity of sensory input to notice it. So, they may need a louder voice, faster movement or stronger smell. Sometimes light touch, e.g. a feather, can help to alert them. Adding in variety can make them notice as well.

Teaching tip

Sometimes when a pupil is not noticing input, it is because they are overloaded (Idea 32). Slow responses and overload can sometimes look the same. It is important to consider the pupil's usual presentation and what has occurred beforehand. This will help you to identify the difference.

Bonus idea ★

It can also help to highlight important information on worksheets for these pupils to help them to know where they need to direct their attention.

Foundations for helping

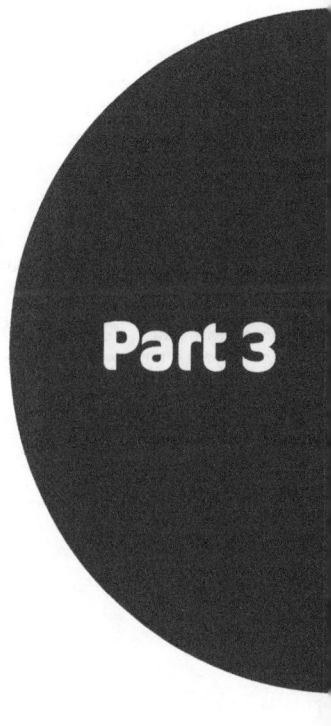

Part 3

What's optimal arousal?

'He always seemed so easily distracted by everything. Like his body was just on high alert, stressed and constantly looking for potential dangers. He just never seemed to be relaxed or calm.'

Arousal at its simplest is how awake or alert you are or how tired you are. Across a typical day, it is very normal for arousal to fluctuate. Pupils, and teachers, need to constantly adjust their arousal levels throughout the day and match their arousal to the task and environment.

It can be helpful to think of arousal like steps or a ladder. At the bottom, you're asleep and at the top you're stressed or highly agitated. Somewhere in the middle you're wakeful and ready to focus on work or play.

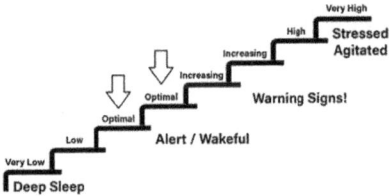

Being able to adjust arousal levels is an important skill. At night-time, pupils need to decrease their level of arousal to go to sleep. At school, they need to maintain high enough arousal to pay attention but not too high that they are overexcited or distracted.

When arousal is too high or low, it is more difficult for pupils to access learning. In order to learn, a pupil needs to be alert or in 'optimal arousal' for learning. The strategies within Part 3 of this book can be used to help increase or decrease a pupil's arousal and get them ready to attend.

Many things impact on arousal level. Firstly, a person's own internal body sensations (Idea 7) give a baseline. If they are tired, their arousal will be lower. If they are hungry, it might be higher or lower depending on the person. The term 'hangry' was invented for those whose arousal increases so they are agitated when hungry! With illness, typically arousal is lower. However, individuals who are unwell have less reserve so they might shift from the bottom of the steps to the top of the steps very quickly. Underlying stress will also have an impact on a person's baseline arousal.

Secondly, different environments have an unwritten expected level of arousal. For example, compare a library, sporting stadium, staff meeting, church, music concert and theatre show. Sensory inputs from the environment also impact an individual's arousal. Each environment gives different sensory inputs. Some people may find a sporting stadium too overwhelming, whereas others might love the energy and noise.

Next, the task or activity impacts arousal. If it is a task the pupil finds easy, it is likely they will be calm. However, if it's a more difficult task, their arousal might increase. Exams are a good example of an activity that can increase arousal. It's also important to remember that arousal can build up over time; each sensory experience will build on the previous one.

Pupils with sensory processing differences usually have more difficulty organising, or regulating, their arousal. For pupils who are more sensitive (Idea 23), sensory inputs from the classroom increase their arousal. This includes everyday inputs like the school bell, pupils singing or the feeling of their glue stick. Pupils can also become quickly overwhelmed by multiple sensory inputs (Idea 32).

Pupils who are slower to process inputs (Idea 26) tend to be more passive. They need additional time to register sensory inputs. Some pupils have a lower baseline arousal but try to actively increase it. They are usually called sensory seekers (Idea 25).

Taking it further

Another thing that can significantly impact arousal and regulation is a previous trauma experience. Typically, the brains of pupils who experience trauma or neglect are wired slightly differently. Their experiences mean that they might be hyper-alert to potential threats or are used to shutting down in order to protect themselves. This means they have even more difficulty organising their arousal, as there are neurological changes in their brain, which makes this harder for them. To read more, look at the attachment resources in the Further reading section of this book.

Sensory strategies

'The terms can be very confusing. I am never quite sure what the differences are.'

It is very important to understand the difference between sensory strategies and sensory integration therapy. Sensory strategies are supports and equipment that draw from sensory integration theory. However, they are different to sensory integration treatment.

Sensory strategies are widely available and frequently used to help to support pupils with sensory differences. They should be monitored to ensure that they are helping with the intended goal. It is important that you are aware of any safety considerations or contraindications for using each strategy.

To take your understanding of sensory strategies even further, please see page 127 for further reading.

A big challenge is that even therapists writing about sensory strategies and sensory integration will interchange the terms. So let's clear up any confusion:

- **Sensory integration theory** is the original theory proposed by Dr A. Jean Ayres. This theory has been built on by other therapists. It explores how the brain processes sensory information to produce a response.
- **Sensory integration treatment** is a specific treatment approach used by trained therapists. Therapists should have completed postgraduate training to use this approach and will be following specific guidelines called a fidelity measure (Idea 31).
- **Sensory strategy** is a solution or equipment that uses the senses and elements of sensory integration theory but does not meet the guidelines for sensory integration treatment.
- **Sensorimotor** relates to movements or activities that use the senses combined with movement. This could include an obstacle course or dance group.

All the suggestions and equipment mentioned in this book are **sensory strategies**, including equipment like ear defenders and weighted blankets, as well as adjustments that you might make to yourself or the environment that help a pupil process sensory information. Though informed by sensory integration theory, they are not the same as sensory integration treatment.

Sensitivity – prepare, advise and warn

'She is so much more organised and focused when I let her know what's happening in advance.'

For pupils who are sensitive, sometimes sensory inputs trigger a fight, flight, freeze response (Idea 12). This response will occur less readily if the pupil has advanced warning of the sensations. This is because their brains will be more prepared for the sensory input and it won't be a complete surprise.

Where possible it's helpful to prepare the pupil for sensory inputs. This can be done with a verbal prompt. It could be a visual reminder or timetable. Video can be a great way to help with preparation. Social stories and sensory stories (Idea 68) can also be used. In some environments the pupil could sit to the side and watch before joining in.

Preparation could include practising in advance. So, for assembly, the pupil might need to spend time in the hall with a teacher, and then with their class, before they go in with the whole school. Alternatively, they might attend for a short period during full assembly before attending for the entire time.

For some pupils, timetables that include the steps of the activity can also be useful. This can help them to know how much longer they need to stay engaged. Using a timer to count down can be helpful for some.

Warning the individual before touch or sounds can help. So, if you are going to touch them to help with something, tell them in advance. If you're going to make a noise (e.g. tipping out a box of LEGO® or ringing a bell), let them know.

Bonus idea ★

For some pupils, the school bell sound or the playground whistle will be difficult. You can help by warning them a minute before it will ring. For pupils who can tell the time, teaching them what time the bell will ring can also help.

Sensitivity – decrease arousal

'The calm space has been a really helpful solution.'

The key thing to remember for pupils who experience sensitivity is that their arousal increases quickly, so they need more support to help their systems calm down.

Teaching tip

Try not to timetable activities that might cause overload back to back. PE, assembly and music typically include extra sensory inputs, and a pupil who is sensitive will cope better if there are breaks between these, and maybe if they are on different days.

Pupils with sensitivity typically have a lower threshold for optimal arousal. As shown on the arousal steps, this means they need less sensory input to increase their arousal. It also means they can be quickly overwhelmed by sensations (Idea 32).

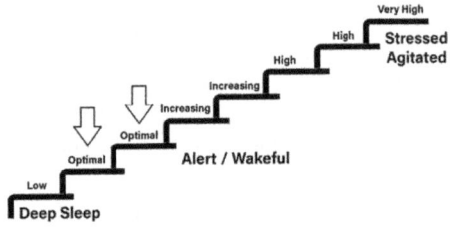

The main thing that helps support these pupils is reducing the overall amount of sensory input they are experiencing. This could include decreasing the noise in the environment (Idea 13) or reducing visual distractions (Idea 40). If there is touch sensitivity, there are extra suggestions in Idea 14.

Bonus idea ★

Strategies like heavy work (Idea 59), breathing (Idea 65) and yoga (Idea 66) can help to reduce arousal. Some pupils find activities like reading, colouring, puzzles or construction helpful. It doesn't always have to be a sensory strategy, just something that helps the individual pupil's arousal.

These pupils also benefit from additional down time to help with regulation. This helps to keep them lower down on the arousal steps! A quiet, calm space (Idea 67) can be helpful at school to support this. When you see the pupil's arousal is increasing, you can direct them to this space. If they find that the noise and movement on the playground add to their overload, they could also access this space at breaks and lunchtimes. Preparing them in advance for sensory inputs is also advised (Idea 23).

Seeking – increase arousal and organise

'I was told that she needs more movement, but the more she moves, the more disorganised she seems to get, so I am at a loss!'

Like pupils who are slower to process sensory information, sensory seekers, or cravers, have a lower baseline level of arousal. But unlike those pupils, sensory seekers actively try to increase their arousal by seeking out more input.

Recent thinking suggests that continued sensory input doesn't necessarily help to organise sensory-seeking pupils. So, they might move and move but never seem to be sated.

The key support these pupils need is organisation and structure. They will need additional sensory input to help to increase their arousal. However, this needs to be provided in a structured way. The structure helps to organise their nervous system.

Look at the sensory input the pupil is craving more of. If it is not helping to organise them (see Idea 27) then think about how you can add more structure to it. You can provide structure using a visual schedule or timer. Rhythm or copying gives structure. A task with steps gives structure. If it's a visual toy or game, turning it on for a short period, then expecting the child to request 'more' gives some structure. Requesting could be done verbally, or with symbols if the child is non-verbal.

For movement seeking you can also try these ideas:

- movement seeking (Idea 16)
- movement minutes (Idea 60)
- sensory diets and circuits (Ideas 61 and Idea 62)
- structured movement (Idea 63).

> **Taking it further**
>
> Read Idea 35: Sensory stims, as the 'seeking' might have a different underlying reason.

> **Bonus idea** ★
>
> For some pupils, puzzles, colour by number or dot-to-dot and visual sequencing activities can be really organising. So, try these as well to see which support is most helpful for the pupil.

Slow – increase arousal

'The slumped shoulders and slowness was an indicator that his body needed to wake up.'

For pupils who are slower to process sensory inputs, their systems need more of the sensory input to register and process it. This usually means they need to experience the sensory input at a greater intensity or for a longer time.

Considering the arousal steps, it takes longer for these pupils to reach optimal arousal. Typically, it takes longer before they are overloaded by the sensation. These pupils can look disengaged and inattentive in class, and they may need extra encouragement to engage in movement activities. Unfortunately, because their behaviour is usually not very disruptive, these pupils are easily overlooked.

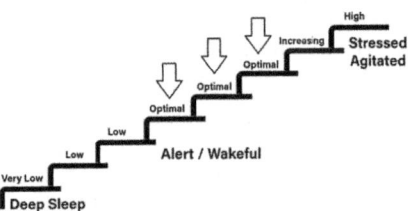

To gain their attention, it can sometimes help if you touch the pupil on the shoulder before giving an instruction and avoid giving instructions from afar. Wait after giving an instruction to allow processing time. If you repeat it straight away, it is another sensory message for their brain to process. Also try:

- low arousal (Idea 49)
- body awareness and personal space (Idea 54)
- posture (Idea 56)
- movement minutes (Idea 60)
- sensory diets and circuits (Idea 61 and Idea 62)
- tactile discrimination (Idea 41 and Idea 42)
- messy play (Idea 43).

Setting goals and monitoring

'I am not really sure why the fidget toy is there. He tends to play with it and this distracts others.'

It is essential that any sensory strategy being used is closely monitored. This includes recommendations that are made by an occupational therapist. Sensory strategies should be supporting the pupil's learning. If they are not then maybe it's not the right solution.

Before you start using a sensory strategy, think about why you're using it. What change do you want to see? At school, goals should focus on facilitating attention, learning and participation. Targets should be set before sensory strategies are tried. Example targets could include:

- increase time spent completing activities or tasks or attending during input
- decrease number of times the pupil needs reminders from the teacher to pay attention
- increase in amount of work the pupil produces or completes
- decrease number of times the pupil engages in a specific activity (e.g. distracting peers, touching others, being out of their chair).

Avoid writing goals or final targets that expect the pupil will be able to manage without their sensory support or equipment, e.g. 'By the end of Year 1 Jon will be able to sit in class without his wobble cushion.' If the sensory support helps, it's because it is giving the pupil's nervous system the sensory input it needs to be successful with attention and learning. Think of it like a pair of glasses. You would never have a goal that the pupil can read without their glasses! Once you have set a target, monitor the pupil for two weeks and record a baseline level of performance. Then implement the sensory strategy and monitor whether the strategy is helping the pupil.

Teaching tip

It is also important to check with the pupil to find out what their views are. Some pupils might not like the strategy, or they may not want to be different from their peers. Where they are able to, make sure you include the pupil in the decision-making.

Classroom set-up

'Once I moved Lily away from Hari she was much more settled and she produced a lot more work.'

In the classroom environment, there are a number of things to think about. It's important to consider not only the individual sensations that activities might have but also which pupils are grouped together.

At first glance, there are some obvious things to consider in the classroom. Are there any distracting sounds? What do the displays look like? But let's dig a little deeper.

If you are going to include movement breaks, yoga or sensory diets in your timetable, where might these occur? Where will you place the calm zone and movement minutes? Perhaps you can use the corridor space or have access to an outdoor space. Some teachers can access the PE hall for sensory circuits each morning.

Next, it's important to consider pupil grouping. Typically, a pupil who is more sensitive will struggle if seated next to a sensory seeker, especially if they have touch sensitivity and the sensory seeker is always in their space. This will put them on high alert. It is important to consider the individual pupil's sensory needs when you're organising classroom groups.

Finally, it is useful to consider how your own appearance and tone of voice can impact on pupils' sensory needs. If you have a pupil with sensitivity to smell, you may want to avoid wearing strong perfumes. If you have a pupil with sensitivity to noise, you may need to consider how the pitch and tone of your voice impacts their listening. For pupils who are easily overloaded, you may need to reduce your own body movements and facial expressions.

Referral to an occupational therapist (OT)

'The occupational therapist was able to provide a full assessment, which included specific guidance and suggestions for us to follow.'

Occupational therapists are health professionals with expertise in both physical and mental health. They help people of all ages overcome the effects of disability caused by illness, ageing or accident so that they can be independent with everyday tasks. This could include basic activities of daily living like dressing or showering or complex activities like driving and returning to work.

Occupational therapists (OTs) may work for the public health services, education, social care or as private practitioners. In the classroom, they can help with functional skills like handwriting, using scissors or participating in PE. At home, they support skills like dressing, feeding and toileting. OTs will also provide equipment like specialist seating, wheelchairs and hand splints.

They can also help pupils with sensory differences. Usually they complete additional training in sensory integration if they are interested in this area. This will include coursework and can include postgraduate training.

Having a basic understanding of SEND and using the strategies in this book will be sufficient for some pupils. For other pupils, assessment by an OT will help to provide greater clarity around their needs. The therapist will also be able to provide specific recommendations.

In the UK, the NHS in the pupil's local area is typically where they can receive support from an OT. Each health authority has a different referral procedure. The school SENDCo is the best person to ask for referral details.

Teaching tip

Parents can usually self-refer to an OT, or school can make the referral. It can be helpful if you write down the concerns you're observing at school to help the parents to know what to say to the therapist.

Taking it further

Some parents may be able to afford assessment by a private OT. In the UK, parents can use the 'find a therapist' feature on the RCOTSS-IP website: https://rcotss-ip.org.uk/.

Referral to other professionals

'There is such a big team around the pupil, and everyone has their own roles.'

Sensory processing disorder is not a formally recognised diagnosis. However, sensory differences typically occur alongside a number of diagnoses including autism, ADHD, Down's syndrome and developmental coordination disorder. For this reason, aside from OTs, the pupil will likely have a number of different professionals involved.

Each geographical area has its own referral process and pathway. You will need to check with your local authority. Your SENDCo should also know how to access each of the professionals. Sometimes parents will be able to self-refer. In some areas schools can make the referral and in other cases it needs to come from a GP.

Roles of the different professionals

Paediatricians are doctors who have completed additional medical training to become specialists in supporting children. The paediatrician is ultimately responsible for making a formal diagnosis, so is often involved quite heavily in the initial stages. They have responsibility for medication prescription and management.

Speech and language therapists are specialists in speech, language and communication. Their role is much broader than just supporting speech pronunciation difficulties or lisps. They have expertise in listening, speaking and social communication.

Physiotherapists support physical development, especially walking and balance. They will likely be involved if a pupil has severe hypermobility.

Educational psychologists are the experts in cognition and learning, with a focus on education. They can make recommendations for reading and learning supports. They can diagnose dyslexia and other specific learning disorders.

Clinical psychologists can also provide recommendations and support for specific learning disorders. In addition, they can assess for a broader range of needs than educational psychologists, such as autism and ADHD. They can also provide counselling and additional family support.

Social workers provide family support and access to additional care resources. Typically there are different teams with different specialities. One team may focus on child protection and another on access to care resources. Some pupils may have more than one social worker.

Behavioural optometrists (orthoptists) are specialist optometrists who can help to support pupils with visual tracking difficulties.

> **Bonus idea** ★
>
> In the UK, local authorities also have specialist teaching services. The teachers in these services have specialist knowledge on specific additional needs (e.g. vision, autism). They are also a great resource to access for advice where relevant.

Sensory integration therapy

'To the untrained eye, sensory integration therapy just looks like play. However, the therapist is constantly adjusting the environment, putting in support to ensure the challenge is just right.'

Sensory integration therapy is a specific treatment approach that has evolved from sensory integration theory. The approach uses a sensory-rich environment, which includes equipment designed to activate the senses, e.g. swings, scooter boards, ball pits, large, soft surfaces and structures to climb on. It is typically delivered by an occupational therapist, but physiotherapists and speech pathologists can also be trained in the approach.

Taking it further

If you are reading journal articles that speak about using sensory integration, you can look to see whether they mention the 'fidelity measure' published by Parnham and colleagues in 2007. This will help you to identify whether they are using Ayres Sensory Integration® or a different approach.

Sensory integration therapy is child-led. The therapist's role is keep the pupil safe and to collaborate on their activity choice. The therapist may adjust the environment or equipment to help the pupil to succeed with their chosen activity. The goal is to provide the pupil with the 'just right challenge' to facilitate an adaptive response. This is when the pupil can complete an activity successfully by adjusting their arousal level, movement and/or plan. During sensory integration therapy, the therapist will always evaluate the space to make sure the challenge fits the pupil's needs.

A typical session will include a mix of proprioceptive, vestibular and tactile-based activities. The types of activities will depend on the pupil's needs: vestibular activities to help with postural control or proprioceptive and touch sensations when there is touch sensitivity. More recently, the term it or ASI® was trademarked to help to differentiate it from other approaches that call themselves sensory integration. ASI® follows the guiding principles set out by Dr A. Jean Ayres when she was developing the model.

Special considerations

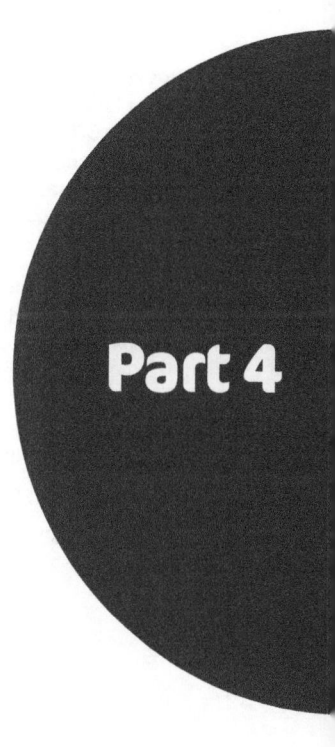

Part 4

Sensory overload and shutdown

'Sam would hide under his desk; this is how we knew he was overloaded and that we needed to give him time to regulate.'

Sensory overload can occur when a pupil's brain has had so much sensory input that it cannot process any more. It can lead to a meltdown (Idea 34) but may also result in shutdown. Shutdown is when the pupil becomes unresponsive due to too much sensory input. It is an internalisation of the overload. Sensory overload is frequently reported in autism.

Teaching tip

You can use a model like the ABC or STAR models (Idea 11) to help to identify what might be triggering overload and meltdowns for the pupil. This will help you to think about and identify patterns and triggers. This helps you to make proactive changes.

It is important to consider all of the sensory inputs that the pupil is processing. We have explored potential classroom sensory inputs in Idea 1. It is important to remember that the pupil will already have experienced sensory inputs at home before arriving at school. They are also processing the internal inputs from their own body.

Sensory inputs are cumulative. So, each builds on the next and the brain needs to process them all. Individuals with sensory sensitivities are typically the ones who experience overload and shutdown. This is because their brains have lower thresholds for the amount of sensory inputs they can tolerate.

Signs of sensory overload are different for every pupil. Some indicators can include going quiet or talking more; an increase or decrease in movement or fidgetiness; a change in skin colour, such as going red or pale; an increase in temperature; a loss of focus or attention; requesting to leave or to know when something will finish; anger, including shouting, lashing out or biting; running away; or hiding.

What to do when a pupil is overloaded

- Make sure all adults supporting the pupil are aware of the signs that the individual is starting to overload. These will be different for each pupil. If you can catch earlier signs, it will be easier to help the pupil to regulate.
- Provide additional downtime through the pupil's day, especially between activities that you know increase the pupil's arousal, e.g. assemblies, lunchtime or a specific lesson.
- Remember that sensory inputs are cumulative. It's like shaking a cola bottle. If you give the bottle one shake, it will probably open without too much spilling. However, if you shake it ten times, it will overflow. Consider the timetable of the day and also how many sensations you are expecting the pupil to process.
- Find activities and strategies that help the pupil to regulate, and include access to these throughout the day. These will be different for every pupil. Some strategies that may help include Snoezelen rooms (Idea 79), massage (Idea 46), breathing (Idea 65) and the strategies listed in Part 7 of this book.
- Consider what other supports, e.g. visual supports, will help the pupil to stay regulated.

What to do when the pupil has shut down

- Reduce demands on the pupil immediately.
- Stop talking.
- Give the pupil time to regulate.
- Take them to a space that they are comfortable with and which has few to no sensations.
- Use a strategy or support with them that you know will help them to regulate.
- Continue to give them time, likely much more than you think is necessary, to regulate and calm down.
- Make a record of what likely caused the shutdown, so you can make changes in the future to help avoid overload and shutdown.

Teaching tip

Ideally, it is important to help the pupil to avoid reaching sensory overload and shut down. The more proactive you can be, rather than reactive, the better.

Bonus idea ★

It is also important to teach the pupil to recognise the signs that they are becoming over aroused so that they can start to independently use strategies. See Idea 87 for more information.

Sensory and autism

'He would spin and flap for hours. It seemed to calm him down. He was really sensitive to sounds and smells as well. Differences in processing sensory information is part of his autism.'

Autism is a lifelong neurodevelopmental condition that affects social communication and engagement. There may be differences in cognition, but this varies. Sensory processing differences were formally identified as a feature of autism in 2013, when the American Psychology Association Diagnostic Manual (DSM-V) was updated.

Teaching tip

When working with individuals who have autism, don't forget visual supports. These could include visual timetables, now and next boards and communication symbols.

Taking it further

Please see the resources in the Further reading section for book and video resources on autism and sensory processing in autism.

Summaries of the literature indicate that 69 to 95 per cent of those with autism report sensory difficulties. Ben-Sasson et al. (2019) have been researching the connection between autism and sensory processing for many years. Their most recent study concluded, like the updated manual, that modulation difficulties are much more likely to occur in individuals who have an autism diagnosis, compared to the general population.

Sensitive, slower and seeking responses are observed in autism. Ben-Sasson et al. (2019) found that scores on sensory sensitivity could be used to differentiate autism from other conditions, such as developmental delays. In addition, the authors found a link between sensory seeking and age, with six- to nine-year-olds scoring higher for sensory seeking. Dyspraxia is thought to occur in between 25 and 90 per cent of pupils with autism (Kirby and Cleaton, 2019).

Supporting sensory in autism

If you are working with an autistic pupil, it is highly likely that you will need to consider their sensory differences. It will be important to determine whether there are any patterns or preferences. An occupational therapist could help with this.

Once you have identified these, you can use the ideas within this book to support the pupil. The exact ideas will depend on the pupil's individual sensory needs.

An additional thing to remember is that the pupil won't only have sensory processing needs. Autistic pupils often need other adjustments to help to support their learning. These should include support from a speech and language therapist. It will also likely include adaptations to the curriculum to match their learning needs.

Fluctuations

Sensory processing differences in autism can fluctuate. Often, they will increase at times of stress and also during illness. In fact, sometimes an increase in sensory behaviours can indicate that the pupil might be becoming ill.

They will also change as the pupil matures. This is normal. Sometimes, an older sensory behaviour may reappear at times of stress or transition. For example, when transitioning to secondary school, the pupil may return to a sensory behaviour that has not been observed for many years.

Sensory stims

Idea 35 covers sensory stimming. These repetitive behaviours are frequently observed in autism.

Overload

Sensory overload or meltdowns can occur more frequently in autism. These occur when the individual has received too much sensory information. See Idea 32 and Idea 34 for more information.

Bonus idea ★

Visual displays, like fish tanks or liquid timers, can be quite calming for some autistic individuals.

Meltdown

'On the outside it looked like a tantrum, but I knew there was a very different trigger and reason for the behaviour.'

People will often describe a meltdown as a tantrum. However, the mechanism is different. Individuals experiencing a meltdown have reached a point of overload. Their nervous system is overloaded and the result is a meltdown.

Meltdowns are an externalisation of sensory overload. They are the opposite of shutdown, which is an internalisation of the overload. Meltdown is typically much more obvious than shutdown.

Meltdowns will look very different for each individual. They may include lashing out, biting, running away, dropping to the floor or shouting. Some pupils may throw things.

In the moment, it is important to ensure the pupil is safe and also to support regulation. The pupil will need time to regulate. Strategies mentioned to support sensory overload in Idea 32 are relevant strategies to support a pupil in meltdown.

When the pupil is regulated, it is useful to create a support plan to help them to avoid meltdown in the future. This will look very different for each pupil. It is important for those supporting the pupil to make sure they are using identified strategies. So, if visual supports help with transitions, these should be used by everyone all the time. If time in the calm zone helps the pupil to regulate before PE, this should be timetabled.

Longer term, it is important that there is a plan in place to support the pupil with their own self-regulation. This is explored further in Idea 87.

Bonus idea ★

The book *The Red Beast: Controlling Anger in Pupils with Asperger's Syndrome* by Kay Al-Ghani is a great story to help pupils to understand meltdowns and also that they can do something to control their feelings.

Sensory stims

'She is always flapping her hands and jumping up and down. Sometimes she seems distressed but sometimes she is excited?'

Stims or stimming is the name given to repetitive movements or sounds that autistic individuals may make. Common stims include hand flapping, repeating sounds and jumping.

In order to support stims, it can helpful to explore why they are occurring, as each reason needs to be supported differently.

Regulation

The individual uses the stim to help with regulation. They may be overloaded (Idea 32) and using the stim to block out sensory information and calm down. In the case of overload, it is important to consider what is causing them to be overloaded (e.g. task, environment). Making changes to this should help to decrease the individual's need to use their stim to regulate. Excitement also increases arousal. I once worked with a pupil who would always flap his hands before dessert as he was so excited about getting ice cream. When exploring this with his mother, she realised that as the stim was safe there was no need to make any changes.

Boredom

The individual is bored and does not have another idea for play. This can frequently occur if the individual has dyspraxia (Idea 10).

Play

The individual enjoys the stim and is doing it because they like how it feels. Some pupils may choose to do their stim in their free play time as it's something they really enjoy. If the stim is safe, then we need to question whether it is really our place to expect the individual to change their preferred play activity.

Teaching tip

Sometimes a stim may be unsafe, e.g. head banging into a wall. In this case, the stim will need to be redirected to a safer alternative, ideally one that provides the same type of sensory input.

Taking it further

There is a growing movement within the autism community towards acceptance of stims. This TED talk, 'Letting Go of Control and Rethinking Support for Autistic Individuals' by Amy Laurent, explores why: www.youtube.com/watch?v=fx3cfzlCG_Q

Biting and hitting peers

'He just keeps biting his peers; sometimes it's when they come into his space but occasionally he will also go over and bite them as well.'

Ninety-nine times out of one hundred, biting or hitting is a form of communication. Your job is to understand what the pupil is trying to communicate. Understanding this will aid you in knowing what you can do to help.

You need to begin with observation. Idea 11 identifies two frameworks (STAR/ABC) you can use to structure your observations. It's important you consider what is happening not only before the pupil bites or hits but afterwards as well, as sometimes the outcome inadvertently encourages the behaviour.

Whilst it is important to support the pupil's sensory needs, some pupils quickly learn that biting or hitting helps them to escape a situation that they are finding overwhelming. It is important to put in place the sensory and communication supports to meet the pupil's needs, alongside appropriate consequences that do not encourage the behaviour to occur.

Every pupil is different, but some common triggers for biting or hitting include:

- Expressing displeasure – this is particularly common in pupils who are non-verbal. They will bite or hit a peer (or adult) to indicate they are not happy (e.g. if a peer takes a toy from them).
- Attempting to engage – for pupils with limited or no verbal language, this might be their attempt to say 'Hi! I'd like to join in!'
- Touch sensitivity (Idea 14) – the pupil will bite or hit as a reflexive reaction when they are touched.

- Sensory overload (Idea 32) – it may be that the pupil who has been hit or bitten was causing the overload for the pupil, or it might be that they are overloaded and the other pupil or adult in their space is just too much to manage.

It is important to request support from a speech therapist to understand the child's level of language. Even for those who are verbal, at times of stress pupils can lose their language, so biting is their communication. The speech therapist will give advice on the best language supports for that pupil.

Use language supports provided by a speech therapist to help the pupil to express their needs. Be consistent and ensure that all staff working with the pupil have been trained and understand how to use the language supports; this includes lunchtime supervisors and any specialist teachers who interact with the pupil. It also helps to teach the other pupils in the class how they can interact with that pupil, especially if they are using sign or symbols.

Look at the structure of the classroom and activities. Consider where overload might be occurring. There might be a pattern in that the biting occurs more frequently at certain times, e.g. playtime. What can be changed at this time to support the pupil? It might be that a specific pupil or adult is a trigger, and this will need to be managed. To avoid overload, use the suggestions in Idea 24 to help to decrease the pupil's arousal.

Finally, it is important to have an appropriate consequence following the behaviour. This will vary depending on the individual pupil's understanding of cause and effect. In some cases, behaviour or sticker charts can help. It is important to ensure the targets on these are very clear. In other cases, a time-out space can be successful.

Teaching tip

Be mindful that the consequence isn't reinforcing the behaviour. For example, if a pupil who is easily overloaded is sent to a quiet space when they bite, they might continue to bite to access the quiet space.

Bonus idea ★

Social stories can be used to help to reinforce the expected behaviour and also consequences if the pupil does bite or hit. See www.carolgraysocialstories.com for more information.

Need for sameness

'She just needed everything to be in the same order each time; if we tried to deviate then it would cause a meltdown.'

Some pupils with sensory processing differences have a preference for order and sameness. For dyspraxic pupils, this can be because they find planning difficult, and leaving things the same requires less planning and organisation. When there is sensitivity, keeping things the same reduces overload and the chance of unfamiliar or difficult sensations. Sometimes, this need for sameness is linked to an autism diagnosis.

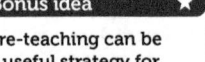

Teaching tip

For some pupils, letting them help to make the changes can be a useful support strategy.

You can help initially by recognising that this need for sameness often occurs as the individual is trying to reduce their overload. At first glance, it can be seen as controlling behaviour. However, framing it this way can cause additional frustration for everyone. Often the underlying need is to reduce sensory overload (Idea 32).

Other supports you can put in place:

- Offer visual supports to indicate changes to timetables or structure.
- Provide warning about changes and when they will occur.
- Give the pupil extra time to process the change.
- Use social stories to explain the change. This can be particularly helpful if resources in the classroom are changing, e.g. if the topic and display boards are changing or the pupil will be moving desk.
- Where possible, a video of the change for the pupil to watch can be a great resource. This is a great strategy for changing classrooms or for school visits. If play resources are changing, you can also make a video of pupils playing with the new resources for the pupil who is struggling to watch and learn from.

Bonus idea ★

Pre-teaching can be a useful strategy for books. For short books, if possible, lend the storybook for the next week to the pupil to read over the weekend. For longer books, ask the parents to start reading the book in advance.

Sensory and ADHD

'It seems that many of the pupils I work with who have ADHD also have different sensory needs. Is it common for them to occur together?'

Research indicates links between sensory processing and ADHD. These include slower responses with the vestibular system and differences with processing touch, visual and auditory sensations.

A review conducted in 2011 reported that sensory processing problems are more common in children with ADHD than in typically developing children (Ghanizadeh, 2011). The reviewers found that sensory functioning had a strong correlation with academic achievement and cognitive processing in ADHD. These reviewers considered multiple articles on the topic. They identified that there were links between ADHD and:

- touch sensitivity (Idea 14), with this being more frequently reported in females with ADHD than males
- balance (Idea 17), with a third of those with ADHD having reduced balance and/or coordination
- auditory processing, including poor directional awareness, distractibility (Idea 13) and slower responses (Idea 20).

Differences with vision (Idea 40) and smell were also reported.

More recently, researchers (such as Isaac et al., 2017) have identified links between the vestibular system (Idea 6) and ADHD. They found that individuals with ADHD have much slower responses to vestibular sensory input than those without. Whilst it is at early stages, this research could help to explain movement seeking (Idea 16) in pupils with ADHD.

Teaching tip

Teachers should be mindful that if a pupil has a diagnosis of ADHD, they may also experience the above challenges with their sensory processing. If you are observing these differences, use the corresponding ideas in this book to support the pupil.

Taking it further

Gabor Maté explores ADHD in more depth in his book *Scattered Minds: A New Look at the Origins and Healing of Attention Deficit Disorder*. Whilst not a specific sensory book, it provides a different perspective on understanding ADHD.

Fussy eaters

'He would only eat a very small repertoire of foods. The foods were all mostly white and dry. He lived off bread, breadsticks and pasta.'

Sensitivity and fussiness with food is another common challenge reported by those with sensory sensitivities. Often, there is a difficulty with textures and sometimes temperatures of food. This is linked to the touch system. Some pupils might also have sensitivity to the smell, taste and look of a food.

Teaching tip

If the pupil is a really restrictive eater, most parents will have tried all the standard advice, so suggesting that they turn the pupil's vegetables into funny faces or make smoothies is typically unhelpful. Start by asking them what they have done first, before giving them any advice.

There is no overnight solution for food fussiness. It is one of the most difficult areas to change and support. Alongside toileting and sleep, feeding is one of the most stressful things parents manage.

Approaches

There are three different approaches that are used to help with restrictive eating. The first is a behavioural approach. For example, the pupil might be told they can't have dessert until they have eaten their meal. The next is flooding, where the pupil is overexposed to the foods they find more challenging until they eat them. This approach can induce a trauma response. The final is a graded sensory desensitisation approach. Here, the pupil is exposed gradually to new foods and textures.

For pupils who have an underlying sensory basis to their restrictive eating, the graded sensory desensitisation approach is, in the first instance, the most effective. Behavioural strategies can be used to help with managing mealtime routines, e.g. it is expected that they sit in their chair, and it is expected that they do not throw food, but the initial approach to eating should be a sensory one. This might be coupled with a behavioural approach in the longer term when you know the pupil is comfortable with the textures.

General tips

- As a general rule, throwing food is NOT OK. Having a scrap plate available for pupils to put food they do not want onto can be a helpful strategy. Make sure this is always the same plate and that it is different from the plates the pupil is using for their food.
- Consider a referral to a dietician to ensure that the pupil is getting enough of the right nutrients.
- There is some very dangerous, unhelpful and costly advice available on the internet, so ensure that parents are interacting with registered professionals and reputable sources. Parents can be very vulnerable and in some cases will try anything that suggests it might help.

Strategies at school

- Some pupils will naturally start to increase their food preferences when they see other pupils eating, and copy their behaviour.
- Have the expectation that the pupil is exposed to different foods, even if they don't eat them.
- The plates with sections can be helpful, as different foods can be on the plate but not touching each other.
- If you have a pupil who is refusing snack time or fruit time, allow them to engage slowly. Expect them to be seated and to be with the group, but let them know they don't have to eat the fruit. It might be that they have their own snack in the group initially. Slowly increase their engagement, e.g. let them pass the fruit bowl around the circle or help to prepare the fruit.
- Messy play (Idea 43) is a good place to start to help with desensitisation.
- Cooking is a great way to increase exposure. Again, expect the pupil to be engaged but don't expect them to eat. Go slowly!
- It may be that the pupil needs to bring a packed lunch. Over time, they might start to eat a favourite school dinner and progress to trying more of the school meals.

Taking it further

The article 'Top 10 myths of mealtime' by Kay Toomey is a useful reference for additional insight: https://sosapproachtofeeding.com/top-10-myths.

The programmes 'Food Train' and 'SOS Approach to Feeding' are specific sensory-based approaches that can support restrictive eaters. They need to be implemented by trained professionals. See https://therapytrain.co.uk/foodtrain and https://sosapproachtofeeding.com for more information.

Visual distractions

'She just keeps looking about and never looks at me. I am not sure whether she is taking anything in.'

Some pupils are very distracted by visual inputs in the classroom. This can draw their attention away from their learning. However, there are some pupils who appear distracted but who are listening the entire time.

Firstly, it is important to consider whether the pupil is paying attention, even if they are not looking towards the teacher. You can do this by asking the pupils questions about the lesson, observing whether they put their hand up or whether they follow instructions when they are given. Some pupils find it hard to look and listen, so they don't look – they just listen.

Other pupils are both not looking and not listening. They won't respond to questions or be able to complete their work after the instructions are given. They will just be thinking about something else. Here are some tips to help these pupils:

- Do not position the pupil near the window or door.
- Consider privacy work screens. Collapsible cardboard ones are easily taken up and down as required.
- Keep the front of the room free from distractions. Make essential information clearly identifiable.
- Colour-coding important information can sometimes help.
- Consider your own classroom displays and boards. How distracting are they? Could you reduce information or have fewer displays?
- Consider only having displays at the back of the room.

Supporting the touch sense

Part 5

Touch awareness – rice/feely bags

'They loved the feely bags. It was a great warm-up activity each morning.'

Pupils with poor touch awareness need additional touch experiences to help them to understand the sensory input they receive from their hands. Removing vision during activities is a way to enhance the pupil's reliance on the touch sense.

Safety

Rice and other legumes are poisonous when eaten raw. These should not be used with pupils who will put them in their mouth.

Rice/lentil/pasta boxes

Finding different items in large boxes full of dry material, e.g. rice, is a great activity to help with touch awareness. Start by hiding large items like toy cars or animals in rice and progress to hiding small items like small beads or counters. Ensure the pupil uses their right and then left hand to find items. Left-handers can start with their left, but don't forget their right hand. Once the pupil can easily find the items, take a cloth and cover the box. Then, the pupil must find items without looking.

Feely bags

Find a pillowcase, or bag of that size, and different-shaped everyday objects. Put the items into the bag and ask the pupil to put their hands in and feel the items, guessing what they are before they take them out of the bag. Initially, pupils will try to cheat and look at the item; make sure they have a guess before pulling it out. Larger, familiar items like toy cars are easier to identify; smaller LEGO® bricks are much harder. You can change the items each day or week depending on the pupil.

Finding your fingers

'When we would sing the finger family song, he could never find his fingers. He would sing but always just raise his thumb.'

Pupils with poor tactile discrimination can have difficulty identifying their fingers and other body parts. This makes it harder to join in with movement songs that require good body awareness. It also means that finger counting is much harder, as these pupils struggle to move one finger at a time.

It is important to help these pupils to find their fingers and body parts. Movement songs, like 'Where is Tom Thumb?', 'The finger family' and 'If you're happy and you know it' are a good start. Pupils with poor tactile discrimination might need extra help finding the body parts. You can use vibration, a brush or touch pressure on the body part or specific finger to help to identify it. If the pupil is not sensitive to touch, you can also use a paintbrush or cotton wool ball.

You can also use messy play (Idea 43) and feely bags (Idea 41) to help with whole hand and finger awareness. Play dough can be used to cover each finger individually. General fine motor activities like tweezers can also be used to help with skills. With these, give each finger a turn, not just the index finger and thumb.

In addition, these pupils often have poor awareness of direction and front and back, so it's important to reinforce these concepts. For example, when playing Simon Says, call out both the front and back of the legs and arms separately. These pupils usually need additional practice when learning connecting parts of the body like the ankles, elbows, knees and shoulders. You may also need to explicitly teach them their individual toes.

Teaching tip

Drawing around hands and toes can help to reinforce the concepts.

Bonus idea ★

Finger puppets are a nice way to isolate the fingers. Just make sure each finger has a turn with the puppet.

Touch sensitivity – messy play

'Her eyes really came to life when we started using the cornflour gloop!'

Messy play is a useful strategy for all sensory modulation subtypes. It is important to be mindful of your goal.

Slower processing and seekers

For these pupils, messy play is a great way to get them engaged. Even older pupils with lower cognition ability usually find messy play enjoyable as it's at their level of ability. It can be a great independent play option. One thing to be mindful of with sensory seekers is that they don't become too highly aroused, so it might be that you need to limit the time or include more structure. An example of structure would be cutting out *six* shapes with play dough or they need to fill *three* buckets with water.

Sensitivity

When there is sensitivity, sensory and messy play can help to increase thresholds. It is important that you never force a touch experience onto a pupil. They must be comfortable. Allow them to have control and progress at their pace. If you're doing something to an individual (e.g. you're brushing them), always ensure you can monitor their responses and give them an opportunity to say stop or ask for more. This may be verbally or with assisted communication, sign or general behaviour. If they pull away or their face or body shows discomfort, it's a clear indication to stop. If they move closer or move your hand back, this indicates that they are comfortable and want more.

Touch pressure

'He just loved hugs, and now I understand touch pressure I understand why.'

The skin has different types of sensory receptors (see Idea 4). It processes light touch and touch pressure differently. Light touch activates a protective response, like if you ran into a spider web. Touch pressure is typically calming; imagine being given a big, firm hug.

Touch pressure can be used to help pupils to regulate. It is also a useful strategy for pupils with touch sensitivity. Typically, this input can help to decrease overall arousal.

Precautions

There are a few necessary precautions:

1. The pupil must feel comfortable with the touch pressure and at all times be able to request the sensory input stops. They should still be easily able to breathe.
2. If you are using your hands to apply pressure, ensure that your fingers are cupped and you're pressing with your palms. Pressing with the fingers can leave marks.
3. Touch pressure should NEVER be used as a restraint technique.

How to apply touch pressure

For younger pupils, touch pressure could be provided with a firm hug. For older pupils, it might be a firm squeeze on the tops of their arms. Sometimes, you can make a sandwich with the pupil lying between two cushions, mats or beanbags. Please use common sense, and ensure you're not squeezing, squashing or hugging too firmly. Make sure you can always monitor the pupil's response.

Teaching tip

The opposite of touch pressure is light touch or tickle. This should be avoided for pupils who have touch sensitivity, as it will increase their arousal.

Bonus idea ★

Brushing (Idea 45), massage (Idea 46) and therapy balls (Idea 73) are other ways to provide touch pressure. Weighted products (Idea 71) and squeeze vests (Idea 72) are both high-tech ways to provide this type of sensory input. In addition, beanbags, and Lycra® tunnels or body bags (Idea 76) can be useful.

Brushing

'I have seen therapists use these surgical-type brushes with pupils but I am never sure what they are for.'

Therapeutic brushing was initially introduced by a therapist named Patricia Wilbarger in the 1990s. It is now referred to as the Deep Pressure and Proprioceptive Technique (DPPT). The technique uses plastic brushes similar to surgical brushes to provide touch pressure and includes joint presses.

General use of the brushes

'Therapressure' brushes or surgical brushes themselves are readily available on sensory websites. Many pupils with touch sensitivity like the sensation they provide. The pupil can use the brush to brush their own skin, or educators can use them. The brushes are designed to be used with some downward pressure. It is recommended that the brushes are only used on arms, hands and legs. If you are brushing a pupil, hold their limb with one hand and brush in a rhythmic manner in the direction of hair growth. Lift at the end of the limb and go back to the top each time. Stay consistent with your pressure and rhythm.

The input should help to calm the pupil. Some pupils like the sensation on their face, but this should always be pupil-, rather than adult-led. Not all pupils like the brushes, and they should NEVER be forced onto a pupil.

Always ask for permission and follow the pupil's lead. NEVER impose or continue with a sensation the pupil doesn't like. Watch for both outward and inward expressions of discomfort. Remember, some pupils might go quiet when they feel uncomfortable.

Taking it further

The specific protocol of DPTT should be taught and monitored by an occupational therapist who has completed the training. The protocol includes brushing the individual's body using a specific technique. It should ideally be administered every two hours. It is not something that can be taught in this book.

Bonus idea ★

To increase a pupil's range of sensory experiences, you can also use other brushes and textures. This could include materials, nail brushes, sponges, make-up brushes, cotton wool, etc. Again, it is essential to monitor the pupil's response.

Massage

'She found the wooden massager on her back really regulating. We used this during carpet time to help her to stay engaged with the lesson.'

Massage is another way to provide touch pressure sensory input. As already mentioned, this type of sensory input can be calming, so it can be used to help the pupil to regulate.

Not all educators will feel comfortable using massage, but it can help some pupils. There are commercially available products that the pupil could use themselves if you do not feel comfortable. You can also teach the pupil to massage their own hands independently.

Before you begin, ask for permission. Only massage the back, hands, arms and legs. As always, it is important to monitor the pupil's responses if you are massaging them and to make sure there is a way for the pupil to communicate 'stop' or 'more'.

You can your own hands or the pupil's hands; commercially available wooden massagers or hand-held massagers with batteries; brushes (Idea 45); or therapy balls (Idea 73).

A quick hand massage for pupils

You can ask your pupils to try this hand massage sequence on themselves. Turn your hands so your palms are facing the ceiling. Put your right hand under your left. Put your right thumb into your left palm and make five circles. Change direction and go the other way. Squeeze your palm and count to five. Push your right thumb up along your little finger five times. Squeeze your little finger. Repeat with your ring, middle, index fingers and thumb. Finish by repeating the palm circles. Then, change hands and repeat.

> **Teaching tip**
>
> This is a great strategy for parents to try at home, especially at bedtime to help the pupil calm down and be ready to sleep.

> **Bonus idea** ★
>
> It can be nice to do the hand massage with moisturiser. Different scents can add variety. Just ensure that the pupil doesn't have any allergies to the ingredients.

Touch and restraint

'The number of times he was restrained was much higher than the other pupils. We realised he was deliberately escalating the situation in order to be restrained.'

This information is only relevant to schools using protocols such as Team Teach, Breakaway or Positive Handling to restrain pupils. If you're not familiar with these, this idea will not be relevant.

Restraint and touch sensitivity

For individuals who are sensitive to touch, being restrained may increase their arousal significantly, resulting in more lashing out or biting. Consider the behaviour plan for these pupils. Reducing contact during restraint or avoiding it may be more helpful, or move the pupil without touching them by creating a half-circle around them and requesting they move.

Seeking-out of restraint

Some pupils like the deep touch pressure that they receive when they are held, so will misbehave in order to be restrained as they find the sensation comforting. This is likely because they find the deep touch pressure input calming. In this case, you will need to set up an alternative form of communication for the pupil to request deep touch pressure, such as using an augmentative and alternative communication (AAC) device, a sign or a Picture Exchange Communication System (PECS)® symbol, depending on the pupil. Staff need to teach the pupil that they can ask for a 'hug' or a 'squeeze' at any time they need it.

Initially, when the pupil requests, it can be helpful to use the restraint hold that the pupil liked. However, over time you can provide different options, including a ball squash (Idea 73) or hug. Some pupils might like weighted products (Idea 71) and Lycra® tunnels (Idea 76) as well.

Touching everything

'He is always touching someone or something. Regardless of where he is sat, he is always fidgeting with something. It can be a bit frustrating for other pupils.'

Pupils with poor proprioceptive awareness typically use their touch sense to compensate. Their proprioceptors don't give them enough information, so they touch things to help their brain to understand where they are in space. When they lean against something, it tells them where their back is. If they are touching something, it tells them where their hands are.

These pupils can frustrate their peers, so sometimes it is helpful to give them extra space beside their desk. It can be helpful to find a fidget toy (Idea 69) if they are constantly touching items on their desk. A weighted lap pad (Idea 71) may also help, as it gives them extra feedback about where their body is.

Before sitting on the carpet, extra movement can be beneficial, as this helps to wake up their system and give them more sensory feedback – try movement minutes (Idea 60) or animal walks (Idea 64). They may also find yoga (Idea 66) and body socks (Idea 76) helpful.

A further consideration for learning disability

Pupils with lower cognitive levels may also continue to touch things because they are still in the sensorimotor stage of development. So, they are still exploring the world through touch and movement. This means they will likely touch and mouth items more frequently than their peers. It is therefore important that all items they are touching are safe to go in their mouth, e.g. toys should be labelled 'suitable for under two years' and paint should be edible. Messy play (Idea 43) is a good strategy for independent play. It is important to consider activities that are at the pupil's cognitive level rather than necessarily their age.

> **Bonus idea** ★
>
> These pupils can also sometimes find the therapressure brushes helpful (Idea 45).

Supporting movement

Part 6

Low arousal

'She seemed to be so slow to get going; once we had her moving and engaged she was great but she needed so much more support to become alert.'

Some pupils will have much lower arousal levels than others. They will need a lot more sensory input and stimulus to increase their alertness and be ready to engage.

Before starting, it is crucial that you ensure the pupil is not overloaded or shut down (Idea 32). Giving more sensory input to pupils who are overloaded or shut down will make them shut down further.

Also, you must always ensure the pupil can indicate for the sensation to stop, or to continue if they want more. For pupils who are non-verbal, you must find a strategy that will allow them to communicate this. It may be you can read their facial expressions. It could be that you stop the sensation and wait for them to move your or their hand back to the sensation.

To help pupils with low arousal, you will need to increase the intensity and variety of sensory inputs. So, if you're using sound, make it louder and add irregular rhythms and beats. Think the opposite of soothing a pupil to sleep. Different visual displays can also help to catch attention.

Light touch or tickle can be a helpful strategy. This strategy must NEVER be used with pupils who are sensitive to touch (Idea 14). A feather, paintbrush or make-up brush can be used to provide a light touch or tickle sensation. Let them explore the textures. If you are tickling, stay on the pupil's hands and arms.

Vestibular sensory input (Idea 6) is also a useful strategy. This sense helps to increase alertness. You could also try swinging (Idea 53), animal walks (Idea 64) or scooter boards (Idea 78).

Dyspraxia – helping ideation

'Angus appeared to have poor attention – he wanted to play but would quickly move on. It all made sense when I realised I had mistaken poor ideation for inattention.'

Ideation is the ability to come up with an idea of what to do. It is the ability to take materials and come up with an idea about what to turn them into. It is the ability to think of a concept for a story or for imaginary play.

Some pupils really struggle to come up with ideas; they will flit between activities because they can't think of how to get started, so they look inattentive. Or, they might not start their work, so they can look like they are unengaged, when actually, they just don't have an idea of what they could write about.

General ideas that can help

- Encourage the pupil to come up with ideas and give them extra time. Sometimes these pupils are great at following along when they are not always challenged to come up with the idea.
- Junk modelling, where you make things out of empty containers, can also be a great way to be creative.
- Follow the leader games, where you have to follow the person at the front of the line, encourage movement ideas.

Tips for creative writing

- Use mind maps to start thinking about different ideas.
- Use prompt sheets with headings, especially for things for like character descriptions, or general outline sheets that ask about environment, beginning, problem and outcome, etc.
- Word sheets with action words, descriptive word and starters for sentences are also great.

Dyspraxia – giving instructions

'I find pupils with dyspraxia are more successful with their learning when I show them as well as tell them.'

A core feature of dyspraxia (Idea 10) is that learning new activities is much more challenging. This is because planning how to do an activity is hard and information is often not generalised from one activity to the next. So, it's like learning each task from scratch, even if only some of the task is new. It could include poor ability to complete the same activity in a new environment.

Taking it further

Work with the pupil's parents to find an extra-curricular activity they are really good at and enjoy. This can help to support their confidence and self-esteem.

To help pupils with dyspraxia to be successful with tasks, you can:

- Give physical demonstrations as well as verbal instructions for new tasks.
- Slow down and repeat instructions.
- Break new activities down into smaller steps and practise each of these first.
- Have a list that outlines the steps for new tasks. Use pictures if the individual can't read.
- Use pre-teaching. This can be really helpful, especially if the family can practise the new activity at home before it is introduced at school. This is really helpful for sports.
- Give the pupil more thinking time.
- Encourage the pupil to think about the plan, especially when you have more time. It doesn't matter if they make errors along the way.
- Give opportunities to use the skills they have learnt. This is extremely important as it helps to boost confidence. For those with dyspraxia, learning new tasks is much harder and often lessons move onto the next concept as soon as the first has been learnt. For an individual with dyspraxia, this means they are always starting from scratch. So, give them a bit more time to *use* the activity they have just mastered!

Dyspraxia – helping planning

'Once I understood that planning was so hard for her, I realised this is where I needed to give more support.'

When helping pupils with dyspraxia (Idea 10), it is important to remember that they don't just struggle to do movements. Before they get to doing, they struggle to think of ideas and plan what they have to do. This could include having difficulty with sequencing, time and organisation.

For those without dyspraxia, planning happens automatically. Information is taken, or generalised, from one activity to the next. The brain uses previous experiences to figure out new ones and to make a guess about possible outcomes. Unless it's a really new or unfamiliar task, much of this happens on autopilot. However, in pupils with dyspraxia, their planning autopilot is broken. You can help them by verbalising your own thought process, so they start to understand the steps. Far too often, these pupils miss out on the planning bit of a task as someone else does it for them. It is really important that they can see the stages and steps of tasks. So, slow down and talk your own thinking out loud. Some general ideas to help with sequencing are:

• making and completing an obstacle course
• sequencing with pictures, including activities, months, seasons, etc.
• following recipes
• LEGO®/construction instructions
• laying the table for lunch
• getting resources out/ready for the class.

Time can also be a challenge for these pupils. This includes larger time concepts, like months, and smaller time concepts, like how long it takes to change for PE. It can help to time activities so that they start to understand time in a practical sense.

Teaching tip

If a pupil hasn't started their work, always double check they know the plan and they know how to get started. For pupils with dyspraxia, even if they have heard the instruction, they still might not be able to figure out the steps of the task or how to get started.

Bonus idea ★

Make sure they have an understanding of the school day, including how long lessons are or how long until home time.

69

Swinging

'The swing immediately helped her to calm down. She would lie on it and we would sing and push with a consistent rhythm and it had a calming effect.'

Swinging is a very powerful sensory strategy. It provides vestibular sensory input. It can be used to both increase and decrease arousal. It's usually something most pupils enjoy doing too.

Teaching tip

Too much swinging can cause overload and can make a pupil feel sick. If a pupil has swung for too long and is feeling sick, heavy work (Idea 59) or proprioceptive sensory input can help them to regulate.

Taking it further

If the pupil is worried about being on the swing, they may have some movement sensitivity. Ensure that their feet are on the ground and they can control the movement until they are comfortable to sit on the swing.

Linear swinging means moving forward and backward or side to side. Linear swinging usually has a calming effect. When the movement is slow and rhythmic, it can be helpful to reduce a pupil's arousal. A song can also be used to help with the rhythm. When it is faster and includes some start/stop movements, it will be more alerting.

Rotatory swinging means spinning around. This type of swinging is usually more alerting. It can be helpful to increase a pupil's arousal. However, it should be used with caution, especially for pupils who are sensitive to movement.

Some schools have swings outdoors for pupils to access. Occasionally, there are swings indoors. If it is identified that this movement helps to regulate the pupil, parents may be able to access a park or have a swing at home so that the pupil can swing before and/or after school to help with their regulation.

Body awareness and personal space

'He was always leaning on the other pupils or had his resources sprawled out all over the desk. Giving him a double desk helped him and the other pupils!'

Pupils with poor proprioceptive awareness typically have poor understanding of where their body is in space. Often they will lean against furniture or other pupils, as this gives them extra touch feedback. This helps them to know where their body is. They can appear quite clumsy and may even trip over their own feet.

Often these pupils benefit from movement with high-intensity proprioceptive sensory input. Examples include:

- swimming
- cycling
- scooter
- trampolines
- walking or hiking (e.g. The Daily Mile).

You can also use heavy work strategies (Idea 59) and additional movement (Idea 60) throughout their day to help to keep their body more alert. Scooter boards (Idea 78) are also a great piece of equipment to help these pupils to understand where their body is.

Some pupils find a weighted blanket or lap pad helpful (Idea 71). This is because it helps to create a barrier around them. It provides extra touch pressure sensory input to help them to know where they are. Marking out a visual space (Idea 55) can also help these pupils to know where to keep their body. They may find leaning against a wall helps with support if they have to sit on the carpet. Also, letting them sit in a chair during carpet time can make it easier for them.

Teaching tip

Allowing these pupils to have more space either side of them at their desk can also reduce the frustration of other pupils sitting next to them. You can achieve this by putting them on the end of tables, or having an extra desk beside them.

Bonus idea ★

Have the pupil trace around their hand and then trace around their whole body. Get them to put their fingernails and knuckles or eyes, nose, belly button, elbows, knees, etc. on the drawings. This helps to improve the spatial awareness of their body.

Marking out space

'The blue circle meant that Stuart knew where to stand. It allowed him to join in the movement group. Without it he would just walk around in between the other pupils or lean on the wall.'

Pupils with poor body awareness and spatial awareness can benefit from a physical marking to outline where they need to be. You can use this physical marking to remind them where to be. Sometimes these pupils struggle with instructions like 'find your own space', so giving them a defined space like a circle can be really helpful.

It can be helpful to use some type of floor marking. In some cases, you may use environmental markers to help to create a boundary. What you use will depend on where you are and what you have.

Classroom carpet time examples

- a carpet square – carpet suppliers usually sell old samples
- a plastic circle or square
- a cushion
- half of a yoga mat
- a classroom mat with an animal, letters or number squares on it – these are great for pupils who need a specific boundary
- a chair if they struggle to stay in their space for carpet time.

PE examples

- a plastic non-slip floor marker
- a mat
- a hula hoop (note these can cause problems for pupils with poor balance as they may trip over the edge)
- a pre-existing marking on the ground, e.g. part of a sports marking
- a piece of equipment, e.g. the football goal
- a physical part of the environment, e.g. a tree or wall.

Posture and core strength

'Isla was always slumped over her table and had such poor endurance.'

Development of good postural control (Idea 17) and core strength should occur naturally as a pupil learns to crawl and then walk. Some pupils have reduced postural control and need extra support to help.

These pupils will typically need more encouragement to join in with physical activity. They may need more support initially, but should definitely be encouraged to join in. Adding endurance or length of time expectations to physical activities is also helpful. Activities that you can encourage in school to help with postural control and endurance for younger pupils include:

- crawling during PE, including commando crawl and on the hands and knees
- scooters/cycling
- climbing up and jumping off PE equipment
- balancing activities in PE and on equipment in the playground
- climbing on equipment in the playground
- obstacle courses in PE
- yoga.

Recommended additional activities for after-school clubs include swimming, cycling, scooters, martial arts, e.g. karate or judo, ballet, gymnastics, yoga and horse riding.

When sitting at their desk, these pupils may benefit from a sloped writing board to help them to sit up straighter. Occasionally, a wobble cushion (Idea 70) can help to increase their arousal when seated. If you have significant concerns regarding the pupil's posture and coordination, a referral to an occupational therapist or physiotherapist may also be relevant.

Taking it further

The online course Sensory Processing with GriffinOT provides additional resources and activities to help with postural control. See www.GriffinOT.com/100ideas.

Bonus idea ★

The Daily Mile is also a great way to get pupils out and walking more. Get your school involved! See www.thedailymile.co.uk.

Bilateral coordination

'Cutting with scissors was such a challenge. Abdu never seemed to be able to organise his left and right hands together.'

Bilateral coordination is the ability to use both sides of the body together in a coordinated manner. This might be doing the same things with legs and arms, like a star jump, or it could be doing a different thing with each side of the body, like when cutting with scissors or using a knife and fork.

Pupils with sensory processing differences, in particular those with vestibular sensory processing challenges, sometimes find coordinating both sides of their body together difficult. They may need support with both gross and fine motor activities. Gross motor activities that can help bilateral coordination include crawling, star jumps, swimming, scissor jumps, climbing, cycling/scooters, dance routines and martial arts, e.g. karate or judo.

The following online resources provide support for gross motor activities:

- The spells in the animation 'Tree Fu Tom' (on BBC iPlayer and CBeebies in the UK) rely heavily on bilateral coordination.
- GoNoodle have great songs to practise body movements: www.gonoodle.com.
- GriffinOT's YouTube channel has a variety of gross motor warm-ups: http://youtube.com/GriffinOT.

For fine motor activities, these pupils often need extra instruction to use equipment like scissors and cutlery correctly. Often, they will cross their hands awkwardly so may need instruction to keep their hands on the correct side. They may need help to put their fingers into the right place on equipment. In some cases, they may also need extra help with postural control first (Idea 56).

Lunchtimes and breaktimes

'We realised that he just needed to get out and move during lunch and breaktimes. Keeping him in meant he was less organised during lesson time.'

For some pupils, lunchtime and breaktimes are the time when they have a natural opportunity to move and refocus. For others, they are extremely overwhelming. It's important to find the right balance for individual pupils.

Sensory seekers and sensory slow

Pupils are sometimes kept in during break times if they don't finish their work or have missed behaviour targets during the day. For pupils with slower responses to sensory input or sensory seekers, this means they miss out on valuable opportunities to move.

It is therefore important that these pupils do not lose out on their break and lunchtimes. These times allow for freedom of movement, which is vital for these pupils. It's a naturally occurring movement break in their school day and one that teachers don't have to scaffold.

Sensory sensitive

For pupils with sensory sensitivities, being out on the playground in larger groups can be quite overwhelming. You may even find that they are frequently in the sick bay, often as an excuse for some quiet time. It can be helpful for these pupils to have a quiet space they can go to at lunchtime, such as the school library or chair outside the school office. Sometimes, pupils might be able to stay in their classroom. The solution will be different for each school but please consider making a suitable quiet space for pupils who are easily overwhelmed by the playground and outdoor space.

> **Teaching tip**
>
> Typically, sensory seekers need to spend more effort focusing and attending to lesson content than others, so break and lunchtimes also offer them the opportunity to have a break from learning.

> **Bonus idea** ★
>
> Lunchtime clubs, like LEGO® club, can also be a great option for pupils who are overwhelmed by the playground.

Sensory
strategies

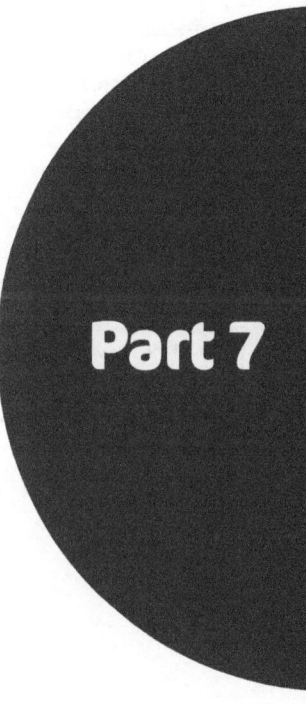

Part 7

Heavy work

'It was amazing how just doing a few press-ups and yoga stretches helped him to refocus and be ready to work.'

Heavy work relates to any activity that activates the proprioceptors. So, anything that involves pushing, pulling, carrying or moving against resistance would be considered heavy work. It is typically used as a calming strategy to support pupils who are overloaded or who need to reorganise.

Taking it further

There is a longer article with more examples of heavy work on the GriffinOT website: www.GriffinOT.com/the-mystery-of-heavy-work.

Heavy work strategies you could use in the classroom include:

- wall press-ups
- regular press-ups
- animal walks (Idea 64)
- carrying a heavy tray, box or backpack (maximum ten per cent of the pupil's weight)
- resistance band exercises
- yoga poses that include weight-bearing like plank, downward dog and warrior poses.

In the playground, you can also consider:

- climbing
- digging in sandpits
- bicycles or scooters
- pulling or pushing old car or tractor tyres
- walking or running up and down inclines
- tug of war
- gardening or forest school.

Bonus idea ★

Having a special heavy book or box that needs to go to the office and back to class when the pupil needs a movement break can be a good solution during the day.

Useful extra-curricular activities to consider include swimming, martial arts, yoga, cycling, rock climbing and hiking.

For pupils in secondary school, age-appropriate activities include weight training, rowing machines and walking on an inclined treadmill. It is helpful to seek advice from a trainer or coach initially.

Movement minutes

'Initially, I found it harder to fit sensory diets into the school day. Movement minutes were a great solution.'

Movement minutes are a simple way to include movement breaks into the structure of the day. All you need is three to five minutes, and you can adapt them to fit the space you have in your classroom. It also helps to do them during lessons when you notice your pupils are drifting off or losing attention.

You can chose three to five of the activities below and do each for one minute. If space allows, you could also make a circular path for pupils to move around the classroom whilst doing the movements. This will depend on your own space.

Movements that easily fit into a classroom space include:

- jogging on the spot
- star jumps
- touching your toes and stretching to the ceiling
- pressing down on your desk and holding
- pressing your hands together and holding
- marching on the spot
- cross-marching – where your left hand touches your right knee then your right hand touches your left knee
- making circles with your arms outstretched
- jumping to the left and then to the right
- twisting to the left and right.

To help pupils to refocus, you can also add in a calming activity at the end. This could include:

- ten breaths
- holding a yoga pose
- sitting with eyes closed for a count of ten.

Teaching tip

See the sensory diet cards page on the GriffinOT website for quick videos pupils can copy: www.GriffinOT.com/sensory-diet-cards-and-videos-free. There are also animations on our YouTube channel: www.youtube.com/c/GriffinOT.

Bonus idea ★

Have a move-it zone for your class. Choose three movement activities each week and put them on the wall for the pupils to follow. Allowing all pupils to access the space creates greater inclusion for those who really need it.

Sensory diets

'I read the term sensory diet on reports all of the time, but I'm really not sure how best to implement them.'

The term sensory diets was introduced by an occupational therapist named Patricia Wilbarger in 1995. Wilbarger proposed that the body needs sensations – to fuel its ability to focus and attend – in the same way that it needs food. Sensory diets should include a variety of sensory strategies to help the pupil to maintain optimal arousal (Idea 21).

Teaching tip

Historically, sensory diets would be very prescriptive, e.g. at 10.00 am John has a movement break. However, sometimes the prescription doesn't match the pupil's current state of arousal. It can be helpful to embed some strategies into the daily timetable and have others to use when you notice the pupil's arousal is too high or low.

Ideally, sensory diets should be written by an occupational therapist following assessment (Idea 29). However, often they are set up in schools using generic advice. A few different books available to support this are listed in the additional materials in the Further reading section. A well-planned sensory diet will offer sensory strategies pupils can use to increase their arousal when it is too low and decrease it when it is too high. Strategies will vary depending on the pupil's needs.

For pupils who need to increase their arousal, movement is often used. Ideas 53, 59–66, 70, 73, 78 and 80 give different examples of movement activities. It is important to consider structure for individuals who seek out movement (Idea 63).

To decrease arousal, calming strategies are typically used. Ideas 32, 45, 46, 59, 64, 66, 67, 71, 72, 75 and 76 all offer examples of calming sensory strategies. Some pupils will find colouring, puzzles, music or reading calming as well.

Bonus idea ★

A portable box, bag or picture key ring with two or three ideas can be helpful for some pupils for when they move to specialist classrooms or for the lunch hall or assembly.

Sensory circuits

'The sensory circuit was a great idea! We did it every morning and at around 2.00 pm when the pupils were losing focus.'

Sensory circuits are a follow on from the idea of a sensory diet (Idea 61). They are essentially like a gym circuit but using sensory-based activities. The goal is to help with the pupil's arousal to prepare them for learning. Usually, sensory circuits are most helpful for sensory seekers (Idea 25) and pupils who are slower to process sensory information (Idea 26).

A sensory circuit will typically include different activity stations. Before setting up your circuit, you need to consider the following questions, as they will help with your planning:

- What space and equipment do you have?
- How much time do you have?
- What is the goal for the pupil's arousal? Does it need to increase, decrease or be organised?

Movement is really helpful for pupils who need to increase their arousal. You can include running, jumping, balancing, catching and throwing – all of the activities you might do for a PE warm-up.

Heavy work or resistance activities (Idea 59) are helpful for pupils who need to decrease their arousal. This could include pushing, pulling and yoga. Lycra® tunnels and bags are also nice to move through. In addition, having a small, dark space to hide in for three to five minutes could be a nice activity to help to lower arousal.

A combination of structured movement (Idea 63) and heavy work (Idea 59) should be considered for sensory seekers. These pupils will typically race around a movement circuit if it is not well organised. Without structure, they may continue to increase their arousal and be less ready for work than when they started!

Teaching tip

The easiest way to include the circuit is to schedule it into your timetable. It might be that a small group of pupils complete it, or it could be something you do with your whole class. Overall, the goal of the sensory circuit is that the pupils will be ready to attend and focus on their lesson.

Structured movement

'She loved singing the song; it helped to reassure her and get her ready to transition to the next lesson.'

Structured movement can help pupils who seek out extra sensory inputs (Idea 25) and also those who find routine and sameness (Idea 37) regulating. This is because it can help to organise their nervous systems.

Teaching tip

Counting the specific number of body movements can also be a great activity to help with one-to-one counting for pupils who find this hard.

Structure can be created in a variety of ways. Using a specific movement song can help with transitions and organisation, particularly for younger pupils and pupils with autism. Go Noodle (see extra materials) has some fantastic movement songs. You may also have a favourite of your own, e.g. 'If you're happy and you know it'. Setting a specific number of movements can help, e.g. do 12 jumps, then run to the door, do 12 star jumps and hop back to your place. This is a sequence of structured movement, rather than the pupil moving aimlessly. Obstacle courses are another good example of structured movement. Rhythm is a great way to add structure, e.g. moving to or copying a beat. It can be done with the body, e.g. clapping and stomping, or with simple instruments.

Simple ball games, like passing a ball around a circle, are a great way to add structure. You can add in more team work by using line games where the pupils stand in a line and pass the ball to the end. The pupil at the end then moves to the front and passing continues until all pupils have had a turn. You can pass the ball through a tunnel if children all open their legs out wide; over their heads; under then over in a sequence; or down the right then left or left then right in sequence.

Bonus idea ★

Follow the leader games also add structure, as the pupil needs to shift their attention and also change movement each time the 'leader' changes.

Animal walks

'Animal walks were a really fun way to include movement throughout the day.'

Animal walks are a simple and fun way to get pupils moving. They involve the pupil taking the posture of different animals, e.g. a bear, a monkey or a frog. The idea is that the pupil will have their body, arms and legs in different positions whilst moving.

The idea with the walks is to add variety to the pupil's movement. Each different animal makes a different position. Some examples include:

- Dog: Pupil moves around on their hands and knees.
- Cat: Pupil moves on hands and knees whilst arching their back up and down.
- Bear: Pupil puts hands onto the ground and walks on hands and feet with their bottom pointing up towards the ceiling.
- Frog: Pupil crouches down on their tiptoes with their knees to the side and fingertips touching the ground. Then they jump up and forwards.
- Crab: Pupil crouches down with their knees to the side and their fingertips touching the ground. Then they move sideways in this position.
- Horse: Pupil gallops like a horse.
- Kangaroo: Pupil jumps forwards with their feet together.
- Snake: Pupil slithers on the floor. (This only works when the floor is clean!)

This list is not exhaustive! You can use a few different walks each time. This activity can be done with or without music. The speed of movement can change, including fast or slow. You can also have the pupils freeze and move on command.

Teaching tip

Twinkl has a number of gross motor animal walk cards if you search on their site: www.twinkl. co.uk.

Bonus idea ★

To add even more variety, have the pupils go backwards and sideways in the positions as well.

Breathing

'We have added in five minutes of breathing in the morning and it really helped to settle the class before lessons.'

Breathing is a really simple way to help with regulation. Slowing breathing down helps to calm the nervous system.

Teaching younger pupils

- Blowing bubbles is a great strategy to start with.
- Use wind instruments like recorders or harmonicas – however, be mindful of sound sensitivity.
- Practise smelling a flower and blowing out a candle.

Supporting older pupils

- Close the eyes and take five or ten deep breaths.
- Rectangle breathing – visualise a rectangle and breathe in for a count of three on the short side of the rectangle, then out for a count of five on the longer side.
- Finger breathing – open one hand and then trace the index finger of the other hand up and down the fingers, breathing in on the up and out on the down.

Online resources

- Moovlee have some great videos for younger pupils on YouTube: www.youtube.com/channel/UCsSS5kMpKCaJ_HhTM9-HKHg.
- Fabelyfy – The Whole Child have some excellent videos for primary pupils, including a 21-day programme: www.youtube.com/channel/UCGYeWtdm9GXYcdgkLph9Rcw.
- The mediation apps listed in Further reading (e.g. Headspace, Smiling Minds) also have breathing sequences.

Yoga

'We started doing ten minutes of yoga each morning and it really helped the pupils to settle.'

Yoga is one activity that can help with self-regulation. There is increasing evidence it can help to reduce stress and anxiety. The positions are also helpful to support postural control and bilateral integration. Many positions can help to improve balance as well.

There are a number of different options to help to engage pupils in yoga:

- Cosmic Kids yoga is a great resource for young pupils. The teacher, Jessie, has designed these videos with pupils in mind. Each video has a storyline that includes yoga sequences. See www.cosmickids.com or find the videos on YouTube.
- Yoga with Adriene is another reputable resource. There are different-length videos. These would be suitable for older pupils who are able to follow instructions. They would be great for a morning or lunchtime yoga group. See www.yogawithadriene.com or find the videos on YouTube.
- Twinkl has some yoga pose cards with pictures and instructions. These could be used in a sequence each week.
- There are also commercially available cards like Yoga Pretzels by Tara Guber and Leah Kalish.
- The book *Sitting Still Like a Frog: Mindfulness Activities* by Eline Snel also includes some suggestions.

For pupils with poor body awareness, this is when they may need a marked-out space to know where to stand. Pupils with dyspraxia might need longer to learn the moves and also more practice with each move.

Teaching tip

Include yoga in your morning schedule so that it is already timetabled in.

Taking it further

In addition to yoga, a number of mindfulness apps are available with meditations for pupils, including Headspace and Smiling Mind. The Scope charity also have a programme called Mindful Monsters. See the Further reading section for details.

Bonus idea ★

A yoga pose is a good addition to the move-it zone as well. See the bonus idea in Idea 60.

Calm space

'We just used a small pop-up tent and added in a few cushions and a blanket. This was a lifesaver.'

For pupils who are easily overloaded, having a calm space they can go to is a useful strategy. This space should be quiet and distraction-free. It should be easily accessible at times when the pupil needs it.

It is important to make sure the space is calming for the pupil. If they find visual inputs overwhelming, try to find a darker or enclosed space. This might be a pop-up tent or it could be under a desk with a sheet over the top of it. If they find noise overwhelming, make sure the space is quiet.

The space will depend on your own classroom and school. Corridors can be helpful, and sometimes the library is used. It is best if this space is close to the classroom, but sometimes this is not possible.

It is important to have support strategies in the space that help the pupil to regulate. Again, these will be different depending on the pupil. Some items to consider include:

- a preferred fidget toy
- a visual timer, lava lamp or bubble tube
- meditation cards or breathing activities
- yoga cards or stretches
- weighted products
- a storybook
- puzzles
- colouring
- construction toys like LEGO® or K'Nex®.

Initially, pupils will need adult support to learn how to use the calm space correctly. Longer term, it should be a space that the pupil can go to and independently self-regulate.

Bonus idea ★

It can be helpful to have a calm box or bag that includes a few of the items the pupil finds helpful to regulate. The box can move to different classrooms with them if they move away from the calm space for lessons.

Sensory stories

'The sensory story really helped to prepare Isla for our trip. It helped to explain to her in advance what it might feel like.'

The term 'sensory story' can be used to refer to two different styles of stories. The first is an interactive sensory story, where readers use extra sensory inputs to bring a storybook to life. The second is when a sensory experience is explained using a social story.

Storybook sensory stories

This style of sensory story is commonly used with pupils who have severe to moderate learning disabilities. It is also a great technique for Early Years classes. The reader enhances the story by adding in sensations.

Typically, everyday objects are used to add sound, visuals, smells, tastes, touch and movement to the story. For example, if the story has a flower then a real flower could be used each time a flower is mentioned, or if there is a drum in the story a real drum can be used each time a drum is mentioned. Typically, a different object will be used to represent each character in the story and characters in the environment.

Social sensory stories

This type of sensory story uses a social story format to explain a sensory experience that the pupil finds difficult. It can also be used to explain what sensations might occur in a new activity. For example, if the pupil needs to have a filling in their tooth, the story might explain the different sounds and touch sensations that could occur at the dentist. If they are going to a firework display, it will explain the sounds and lights.

Teaching tip

Twinkl has a number of pre-written sensory stories available to members.

Taking it further

This video, 'Making play inclusive – sensory stories' by Sense Charity, explains how to turn a storybook into a sensory story: www.youtube.com/watch?v=BzaU-PCvTZM. To learn more about social stories visit Carol Gray's website: https://carolgraysocialstories.com.

Sensory
equipment

Part 8

Fidget toys

'The sticky tack worked a trick; it really helped her to focus and maintain her attention.'

Sensory fidget toys (also known as sensory fiddle toys) can be a useful solution for pupils who are constantly fiddling at their desk. For some, a fidget toy might just mean the difference between concentrating and attending to what the teacher is saying or missing much of the lesson. They don't work for every pupil and in some cases can cause more of a distraction!

For some pupils, fidgeting or fiddling with something helps to sharpen their attention. Often, they will play with anything that is on their desk. The goal of a fidget toy is to give the pupil a more appropriate and less distracting item to fiddle with.

It is important to choose a toy that is silent and will not distract other pupils in the classroom. It's useful to find one that is robust as well. Some examples of everyday objects you could use include:

- sticky tack
- a small piece of fabric
- a keyring
- a LEGO® piece or person
- a rubber snake toy
- a stress ball.

Commercially available products include:

- tangles
- stretchy men
- koosh balls
- twist and lock blocks
- theraputty.

Wobble wobble wobble

'The wobble cushion really helped him to stop rocking in his chair and reduced the number of times that he stood to approach me during the day.'

Air-filled 'wobble' cushions are a staple in most SEND departments. These cushions are typically disc- or wedge-shaped and are designed to be filled with air. They should provide an unstable surface for the pupil to sit on as an alternative way for them to fidget.

For the pupils they help, wobble cushions can be a great, and inexpensive, strategy. They are, however, not a one-size-fits-all solution. Some pupils really dislike the feeling of the cushion. Others get tired because of the extra effort it takes to sit on the cushion. And, for some, they don't make any difference.

Wobble cushions are primarily designed for movement seekers but can sometimes help pupils who are slower to process movement. Pupils who may benefit from a wobble cushion include:

- those who are rocking in their chair
- those who frequently move about in their seat or constantly approach the teacher
- those who are slumped over, struggling to focus.

Wobble cushions must be inflated so that when the pupil sits on them the base remains flat, but there is some movement in the cushion itself. If there is too much air, the base will be very unstable, and if there is too little, the cushion won't provide any movement. It is essential that the pupil's feet still touch the floor when they are sitting on the cushion.

Teaching tip

It is expected that the pupil will move about on the cushion. Their movement should be less distracting to the class and safer than rocking back on their chair. If the cushion is making them more distracted or more of a distraction, then it is not the correct strategy for that pupil.

Taking it further

Sit on the cushion yourself. What's your first impression? Do you like the feeling of sitting on it? Not everyone likes the feeling and it's useful to know what your pupils are experiencing when they sit on the cushion.

Weighted products

'The weighted blanket was a really good addition to our calm space.'

Weighted products come in all different shapes and sizes; there are blankets, vests, lap pads, shoulder pads and stuffed animals. They are usually recommended by occupational therapists. They are frequently seen in special schools and some SEND departments will have them available.

The core idea behind weighted products is that they give additional touch pressure. If the pupil or adult is moving under them or carrying them, they also provide additional proprioceptive sensory input.

Safety

There is a general rule that weighted products should weigh no more than ten per cent of the pupil's body weight. It is essential that pupils are always monitored when using weighted products, especially weighted blankets. **These products are not toys**. Unfortunately, there was a well-documented case in Canada where a pupil died after being rolled up in a weighted blanket and left unsupervised. The blanket restricted their breathing and they suffocated.

Choosing a product

Designs with pockets for the weights are recommended. This ensures that the weights stay evenly distributed in the blanket or lap pad. For the interior, plastic poly pellets or glass pellets are better options than sand or rice. You must also consider how you will wash the product, which will need doing at some stage. The stuffed animals are much harder to clean, if they are being shared between pupils. Many blankets and lap pads have a fire-retardant, easy-clean surface, which is often much easier to manage in schools. For larger products, being able to remove the weights can be helpful for your washing machine. Also, it can allow you to change the weight for different pupils. However, if your pupils will play with the weights and try to remove them, then sewn-in weights may be a better option.

Weighted lap pads and stuffed animals

Weighted lap pads and stuffed animals are designed to sit on top of a pupil's lap. These can be great for pupils who have poor proprioceptive awareness, as it gives them extra feedback about where they are. This can decrease their fidgeting and also help them to stay in their space, especially on the floor. They can also be used with small pupils instead of a blanket when lying down.

Weighted shoulder pads

Weighted shoulder pads are designed to sit on the pupil's shoulders. Some pupils don't like the feel of the pad on their neck. The snake-shaped stuffed animals can sometimes work better, as they conform around the neck and shoulders. Larger lap pads can also be folded in half long-ways and draped over the shoulders for the same effect.

Weighted vests

Weighted vests are designed to be worn over the top of clothing. They usually work better than shoulder pads as they don't fall off. Usually, you can adjust the weight to suit the needs of the pupil.

Weighted blankets

Weighted blankets are much larger than lap pads. They can be purchased in single and double bed sizes. It's important to monitor pupils closely when using weighted blankets. Always ensure you can see the pupil's face and monitor their breathing. Only allow them to put their face under the blanket if they are independently able to move out from under it and can verbally respond that they are OK. NEVER leave the pupil alone under the blanket. Weighted blankets can work really well for some pupils, but there are risks associated with using them. If using them in a school, make sure there is a clear policy in use and all staff are aware of the risks.

> **Bonus idea** ★
>
> For pupils with poor body awareness, you can put soft toys under a weighted blanket and ask them to go under and find and collect them.

Tight clothing and squeeze vests

'He was always much calmer at the beach when he was wearing his wetsuit. We realised this was because of the additional pressure it gave on his skin. Using hug-shirts was a great option for under his school uniform as it gave the same sensation.'

As previously mentioned in Idea 44, touch pressure is calming. There are a number of commercially available products that aim to provide touch pressure for pupils throughout the day. These are usually recommended by occupational therapists and purchased by parents. Special schools will sometimes have neoprene vests to use with their pupils.

Teaching tip

Expensive products like squeeze vests should be rented or trialled before a purchase is made.

At the lower tech end, there are t-shirts designed to give additional touch pressure, like the 'sens-ational hug tee'. These are designed to be worn under clothing. This can be problematic in warmer weather. Some families use off-the-shelf products instead of specially designed options. A slightly small t-shirt can give the same effect. Swimming rash guards and bicycle shorts provide a similar type of touch pressure, as do tights with a higher amount of elasticity. Next, there are products made from neoprene that are designed to be worn tightly over the top of a school uniform, such as the 'Bear Hug' by Southpaw. These usually wrap around the pupil's torso and have straps that go over the shoulders. Typically, they are secured together with Velcro®, and can be adjusted to fit the pupil's body size. They can be worn for periods during the day and easily put on and taken off. At the high-tech end, there are 'squeeze vests'. They are vests that the pupil can inflate and deflate with air as required. They are similar to a scuba-diving buoyancy control device. When inflated, the vest gives the pupil's body a big squeeze.

Bonus idea ★

Taking the neoprene vests off is a good activity to provide the pupil with extra proprioceptive input, as the pupil needs to pull strongly on the Velcro® attachments to remove the vest.

Therapy balls

'We used the big ball to provide touch pressure, like a massage. It was a great way to do this for our older pupils.'

Therapy balls or large gym/Pilates balls are inexpensive pieces of equipment that can be used in a variety of ways. They are a great tool for squashing and are also good to help with balance and postural control.

A note on size

The balls come in a variety of sizes. A 55 cm ball will be more suitable for pupils under five years of age and 65 cm is most flexible for older pupils. However, you must consider the pupil's height. If using the ball to sit on, the pupil's feet should firmly touch the floor when they sit on the ball. Their knees should be just below their hips (between 90 and 120 degrees).

Using for balance

For pupils with very poor balance, just sitting on the ball might be a challenge for them. Deflating the ball slightly makes it more stable than if it is fully inflated. Pupils can then sit on the ball and march their feet. Next, they can try to softly bounce on the ball. Finally, they can try to lift one foot off the ground and balance on one foot. As an extra challenge, they can try to touch their hand to the opposite foot when it is lifted.

Using for touch pressure

The balls can be used to provide touch pressure. Have the pupil lie on a mat then roll the ball over the top of them. Roll with a firm consistent pressure and speed. Avoid the genital area and head. If the pupil puts their arms and legs out like a starfish, they can direct where they want the ball to be rolled.

Teaching tip

Never force the pupil to engage in any of these activities if they feel uncomfortable.

Bonus idea ★

The ball is a great option for heavy work. If an adult holds the ball, the pupil can push against it with their hands. The pushing provides extra proprioceptive sensory input.

Vibration

'He really liked the vibrating cushion – it seemed to really calm him down.'

Vibration can be a useful tool for some individuals. This sensation is carried by the touch sense and in some cases can be very regulating. It can be a great way to engage individuals who are slower to respond to sensory input.

Different products

There are a variety of products available. When searching, it is best to stick to sensory product sites, as searching for 'vibrating toy/s' will provide you with interesting search results! Products include:

- cushions for sitting on/putting feet on
- longer snake-like tubes
- toys for the mouth like the Z-Vibe
- hand-held massagers (also commercially available)
- vibrating gym plates.

Trouble-shooting

Some pupils don't like the noise that vibrating products make. You can help by allowing them control of the on/off switch so they can see where the noise comes from.

How to use

The pupil must have control. If you're putting the items on the pupil, look for indicators they want more. Always make sure they can ask you to stop, whether verbally or non-verbally. If you're behind the pupil, sitting in front of a mirror can help you to see their face and monitor for a response. Start with the pupil's hands and arms, then move to their back and legs. Some pupils will like the feeling of vibration on their face but avoid this for pupils with epilepsy, as it may cause a seizure.

Chew toys

'She was always chewing on her collar. Once we got the sensory chew, this reduced and she seemed much calmer.'

Sensory chew toys can be a helpful strategy for some pupils. However, choosing a sensory chew toy for a pupil can be a daunting task. There are so many different ones available!

Before you begin, consider the reasons a pupil may chew. These are explored in Idea 18. Each pupil should have their own allocated chew toy. These should be cleaned daily, following the manufacturer's instructions.

Consider where and how the pupil chews

'Where' refers to 'where in the mouth'. Have a look at how the pupil chews. Pupils who chew or suck at the front may prefer a rounder chew. If they chew on their back teeth, a longer toy, such as a P or X shape, will be better. Also consider how hard they chew. If the pupil chews really hard, they will need a tougher chew but if they suck, a softer one might give them more feedback.

What texture and shape do they prefer?

Start with what the pupil currently chews. This will help you to understand their preferences, e.g. fabric is a very different texture to a piece of LEGO®. If they chew fabric, they may prefer a bandana. If they chew items with texture, a chew toy with patterns might be preferred.

Is a sensory chew toy age- or socially appropriate for the pupil?

For pupils with significant learning disabilities, a sensory chew toy may be appropriate. For pupils in mainstream school with a high level of social awareness, a chew may not be appropriate. Pencil toppers and 'chewlry' are less obvious alternatives or try sugar-free chewing gum if policy allows.

Teaching tip

Ensure the pupil is not being distracted by their toy, zoning out or being a distraction to others. The chew toy should be used as an alternative to chewing something else and should be helping with attention and participation.

Bonus idea ★

A container on their desk to store the toy when they are not using it can help with hygiene.

Stretchy tunnels and body socks

'The Lycra® body sock doubled as a calm space. He found it really regulating going inside and taking some quiet time.'

There are a few different tunnels and body socks/bags commercially available. These are typically made from Lycra® material. They give additional touch pressure when the pupil moves through or inside them. They can be used to help with regulation and also body awareness.

Most sensory equipment retailers have a version of a Lycra® tunnel and or/sock. The tunnels are a long piece of tubular material that pupils can go inside and crawl through. The socks are usually a rectangle shape with an opening in the middle for the pupil to go inside.

An easy way to make a tunnel is to purchase tubular knit fabric from a fabric shop. This comes pre-woven in a tunnel shape. If you have the skills, you can also sew one from Lycra® or knit material.

When using them for regulation, usually the pupil will go inside and treat it as a quiet space. Some pupils like to sit inside the socks at their desk, as the extra touch pressure helps them to regulate. They can also stretch out inside the sock to receive even more touch pressure and some proprioceptive sensory input.

Pupils with poor body awareness or movement sensitivity sometimes do not like being inside these products as they can't see what's happening. If so, proceed very slowly. Play hide and seek, putting just your head inside whilst sitting down. Allow the pupil to come in and out in a playful way. Never force them to be inside and always make sure they can easily get out.

IDEA 77

Ear defenders

'We used the ear defenders during assembly and lunchtimes as they really helped Ravi to stay in the space and engage.'

Ear defenders, or noise-blocking headphones, are a common piece of sensory equipment. They can be helpful for pupils who are sensitive to sounds. They are readily available commercially.

The available products are all similar price points, and you will easily be able to find them in sensory catalogues and general suppliers (e.g. Amazon). Some pupils prefer ear plugs over ear defenders. Ear defenders won't work for all pupils, as some pupils don't like wearing them because they muffle sounds.

Typically, pupils will use the ear defenders during noisier periods. This might be during music lessons or assembly or when in the lunch hall. Sometimes, pupils will wear them when they need to sit and focus on work. Other pupils will use them when their classmates start to become louder.

The pupil should be reasonably independent in putting these on and taking them off. Some pupils might need a reminder to put them on. Other pupils will independently decide when they will use them.

More recently, noise-cancelling headphones have started to be used by some pupils. These can be expensive, and typically parents have purchased them. The noise-cancelling feature can be used with or without music playing.

Teaching tip

Teach the pupil to access the headphones when they need them. Have them freely available for the pupil to access and put on and take off.

Bonus idea ★

For pupils with larger heads, sometimes gardening noise protection headphones are more comfortable as these come in adult sizes.

Scooter boards

'The scooter board was a really fun way to help the pupils to increase their endurance and postural control.'

Scooter boards are square or rectangular boards with four wheels on the bottom. They look a bit like skateboards. They are a great tool to help to support endurance and postural control. They can also help with regulation.

Safety

Whilst these look like skateboards, scooter boards should NEVER be stood on. They move very quickly and will roll out from under the pupil. This usually results in the pupil falling and potentially hurting themselves.

Type of sensory input

Scooter boards provide both vestibular and proprioceptive sensory input. The vestibular input comes from the movement. The proprioceptive input comes from the pushing the pupil needs to do to move the board.

How to use

The pupil should lie on their stomach and use their hands to move the board forwards or backwards. When used maturely, the pupil should balance on their stomach, with their legs stretched out so their feet are off the floor. Then they propel the board by pushing with their hands.

A harder challenge is to lie on the back and propel the board with the feet. The board will move backwards. The pupil must keep their head off the ground by curling their chin to their chest.

Scooter boards can be used in sensory circuits (Idea 62) or as part of a sensory diet (Idea 61). They should help to organise the pupil to be ready to work. Some pupils will become over-alert from the movement, and in this case it's not the best solution.

Snoezelen (sensory) rooms

'These rooms always look so impressive! With their bubble tubes, disco balls, music and fibre optic lights, they seem to help some pupils to really calm down.'

Snoezelen – or sensory – rooms are the rooms with lights, bubble tubes, music and sometimes vibrating surfaces. The goal of these rooms is to create a relaxing space that helps to reduce agitation and anxiety. The spaces can facilitate relaxation and development, provide stimulation and be used for therapy. They can also be used to engage the pupil, stimulate reactions and encourage communication.

These rooms can be used in a variety of ways. Each room will have different equipment. If you are not sure how to use the equipment, check with your therapist or the company that installed the room.

It is essential that you have set goals (Idea 27) before using the room. Goals could include:

- regulation and calming
- interaction and turn-taking
- choosing
- teaching children to use switches.

If the goal is regulation, then it is important to find the equipment that helps the pupil to regulate. This will be different for different pupils. The same piece of equipment won't work for every pupil.

The spaces can be used to support therapy outcomes, especially joint attention, choosing and switch use. This could include understanding cause and effect and also waiting. You can use switches to support attention, choosing and language. For example, switching the bubble tube on and off before passing it to your partner is a great turn-taking game. You can use equipment that the pupil is motivated by to support PECS® exchange.

Taking it further

The book *Multiple Multi-Sensory Rooms: Myth Busting the Magic* by Joanna Grace explores tips and strategies for using these rooms.

Bonus idea ★

If you have a UV light, whiteboards and UV pens can be a great way to support mark-making and writing. A lot of pupils find this quite fun, and they also sometimes find it easier to look and focus on their drawing as the room is otherwise dark and free from distractions.

Creativity in playgrounds and PE

'It doesn't always need to be a piece of special sensory equipment. Make sure you have a look at the existing resources you have in your school too.'

If you have a look around your school, you will find all sorts of sensory equipment. Sometimes it's useful to think outside the specialist equipment catalogues and have a look at what is already there.

First, have a look at the playground. Is there a trim trail? This is a great place for heavy work and for a sensory circuit. Is there a climbing net or frame? This is another piece of equipment that provides huge amounts of proprioceptive sensory input. Are there any balance steps or beams? These can help to support the vestibular sense to develop.

Next, what's in the PE cupboard? Skipping ropes make great tug of war ropes. Hoops and spots can be used for jumping and as markers for movement. Is there any climbing equipment? Or any equipment you can jump over or off? All of these can be used to increase vestibular and proprioceptive sensory input.

Some schools are fortunate to have soft play areas – or at least some soft play pieces. These are fantastic for encouraging movement and motor planning. Barrels can be used to help with movement sensitivity; just make sure you use them slowly. Blocks can be used for building, which helps planning and is a great form of heavy work. Ramps and steps are also a great way to increase proprioceptive sensory input. And, if you don't have a soft ramp, a sloped part of the playground is a good substitute.

Functional skills

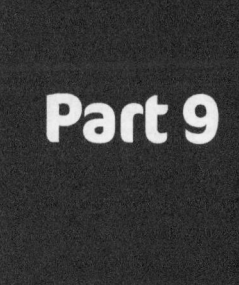

Part 9

Won't hold a pencil

'She avoided the pencils with grooves but we realised it was the feel of them. Once we gave her smooth pencils she was happy colouring and mark-making!'

Difficulty holding a pencil can occur for a number of reasons. Sometimes a pupil might not have the fine motor skill maturity to grasp the pencil. Some pupils don't like the feeling of specific pencils. Others have a really loose or tight grasp. This idea explores each of these.

Taking it further

This page provides video reviews of common pencil grasps: www.GriffinOT.com/pencil-grip-reviews.

Bonus idea ★

Pencil grips can sometimes be a solution. Cylindrical grips come in different textures, and the pupil may prefer the feeling of these in comparison to the wood feeling of the pencil. They may also prefer pens with grips on them when they are older. Softer pencil grips, which give a little bit of feedback, may help those with both tight and loose grips.

Immature fine motor skills

Pupils with immature skills will need more time to develop their fine motor skills. Take a step back and encourage them to engage with general fine motor activities like play dough, beading, LEGO® and craft. Messy play (Idea 43) and rice/feely bags (Idea 41) can also help. The pupil may also find finger crayons easier to hold.

The feeling

When the problem is the feeling of the pencil, this is 100 per cent linked to the touch sense. You can try different types of pencils, as some have a smoother finish. Also, some pupils might prefer round-shaped pencils, as these do not have any grooves on them.

Loose or tight grasps

Difficulty with grasp pressure is linked to proprioceptive awareness. Individuals with loose grasps sometimes need more support to develop their fine motor skills. They may also find thicker pencils easier to manage than thinner ones. For pupils with a tight grip, you can also try a mechanical pencil. When the pupil uses too much force, the lead will break. This can be quite frustrating, so will only work for some pupils.

Handwriting

'She found handwriting really tricky, especially when we switched to cursive. It was really hard for her to organise and plan her letter formations.'

Handwriting is a skill that pupils with dyspraxia often find more challenging to learn. Difficulties with visual perception or interpreting the direction, size and space of what you see can also impact on handwriting.

Handwriting is a very complex skill. It requires not only good sensory awareness and motor skills, but also adequate memory, cognition and language. Each area needs to be considered.

When there is reduced touch and proprioceptive awareness, it can be harder for the pupil to feel and organise the direction of letters. You can use multi-sensory approaches to help, such as drawing in sand or shaving foam. You could also try asking pupils to trace letters on sandpaper and textured letters.

Pupils can also benefit from feeling letters to understand their shape. Put wooden letters into a feely bag (Idea 41) for them to identify. Alternatively, draw letters on their back for them to guess.

When there is dyspraxia, it can be harder for the pupil to learn the letters initially. It is important to:

- Give these pupils more instruction and time when they are initially learning their letters.
- Make sure they have their letter formations correct.
- Consider teaching letters in letter formation groups rather than phonics groups. The letter formation families are as follows: ltij; rnmhbp; uy; coadgq; vwkxz; and fse.

Taking it further

There are further ideas to support handwriting on the GriffinOT website: www.griffinot.com/category/handwriting. The National Handwriting Association have a number of resources on teaching and supporting handwriting, including training: https://nha-handwriting.org.uk.

Bonus idea ★

When the pupil uses a tablet for letter practice, give them a stylus to hold so they can also practise their pencil grip.

Cutlery use

'He cut so forcefully that the food would fly off his plate.'

Using a knife and fork relies on both planning and bilateral coordination. The proprioceptors in our hands also make sure that the pressure used is correct – too little and the knife won't cut, too much and food will fly off the plate.

The only way to improve cutlery use is to practise and have the expectation that cutlery will be used at mealtimes. Some pupils will need explicit instruction for the different steps of cutlery use, including:

- where to put their index finger
- how to curl their little, ring and middle fingers around the knife and fork
- how to hold their fork steady whilst sawing with their knife
- how to saw back and forth with their knife
- putting their fork into the food at the cutting end (i.e. left side)
- cutting on the right side of the fork, so that the cut piece of food ends up on the fork
- putting soft food on first before harder food so multiple foods can go onto the fork
- how to scoop small items, e.g. peas, onto the fork with their knife.

Cutlery use can be practised with play dough, including making pretend sausages. Then, it's best to practise at meal times. Start with softer food, which is easier to cut, and progress to harder foods.

Additional tips

- Shorter children's cutlery is easier to manage initially than adult-sized knives and forks.
- Thicker handles can help pupils who have loose grips.
- Cutlery with marked holes for the index finger can help some pupils.

Difficulty on playground equipment

'She almost seemed scared of the swing and the slide. She never went on them.'

Using playground equipment requires good balance and coordination. It is much harder for pupils with poor vestibular awareness and dyspraxia. For those with vestibular sensitivity, it is also scary, as they can feel uncomfortable when their feet are off the ground.

Firstly, you need to determine whether the pupil is avoiding playground equipment because they can't figure out how to use it or whether if they are uncomfortable with movement. Those who are unable to figure it out will likely avoid everything, until they are shown. If it's a movement problem, the pupil might avoid equipment that is high or moves a lot but play on more stable equipment.

Supporting planning

- Pupils with dyspraxia will likely need to be shown exactly how to use playground equipment and may need new instructions if they move into a new playground.
- They will need more practice using the equipment to feel comfortable.
- They may find it easier to become confident on equipment when the playground is emptier. So, perhaps time before or after school could be arranged for them to practise.

Supporting movement sensitivity

- These pupils need to be allowed to progress at their own pace.
- They will find equipment where their feet still touch the ground easier than equipment where their feet are off the ground.
- Using the equipment when the playground is quieter is likely to be easier for them.

Teaching tip

Some pupils gain confidence by watching others. It may help to have a buddy for the pupil to watch and then follow, especially if the buddy can also help them during break and playtimes.

Taking it further

A referral to an occupational therapist could help those with movement sensitivity.

Bonus idea ★

Consider the suggestions for dyspraxia in Ideas 50 to 52 as well.

Body awareness and counting

'Her one-to-one correspondence is really poor. She can't count on her fingers or with counters.'

Sometimes when pupils struggle with one-to-one correspondence, it is because they have such poor body awareness that they can't link their voice, or counting, to their body. These pupils need more practice coordinating the two.

The easiest way to do this is with bigger movements first. These pupils are likely to struggle coordinating movement actions with their voice alongside counting. They will also probably have difficulty with rhythm. Try the following activities to start with:

- clapping and saying 'clap' each time the hands come together
- drumming and saying the word 'bang'
- stomping with the feet, coordinating this with the word 'stomp'
- jumping feet apart, then feet together, coordinating 'open' and 'close' with the movement.

This list is not exhaustive. The goal of the activities is for the pupil to coordinate the movement with the word. Once the pupils can do a basic beat, change the speed and rhythm.

Next, the pupil needs to practise moving and counting at the same time. Many pupils with poor body awareness find it hard to count in time with their movement. Ask the pupil to do an activity a specific number of times and then stop. For example, 'Can you do six jumps?' Count with the pupil and make sure they stop on six. Make sure they count each time their feet touch the ground. The goal is that the pupil counts correctly and stops correctly each time. If they don't, they must start again! Most pupils like this game.

Poor attention in class

'He missed so much of his learning as he just wasn't paying attention.'

Difficulty with attention is not uncommon in pupils with sensory differences. It can occur for many reasons. Sometimes it is due to low arousal. Sometimes it is linked to overload. And, in some cases, it's linked to distractibility.

Firstly, it is important to double check whether the pupil is actually attending. Some pupils may be showing poor visual attention but may actually be engaged. You can monitor this by asking them questions and looking to see whether they follow your instructions without an additional prompt.

For pupils who clearly aren't paying attention, the next step is to identify why this might be. If they are slower to respond and appear disengaged, then Ideas 51, 55, 62, 63 and 64 may help to increase their arousal. Equipment like wobble cushions (Idea 70) and fidget toys (Idea 69) can sometimes help.

If they are visually distracted, Idea 40 lists additional strategies. It may also be that they are distracted by sounds. If this is the case, the ideas for sound sensitivity may help (Idea 13).

In addition, some pupils with touch sensitivity (Idea 14) also have poor attention in class. This is because they are constantly being distracted by the small touch sensations from their clothing, or maybe a breeze or their peer brushing past them. Their attention is then drawn to these sensory inputs rather than the teacher's lesson.

Teaching tip

It may also be that the pupil has ADHD, in which case a referral to a paediatrician would be the next step.

Sensory and emotional regulation

'We have been using the Zones with the whole class and have found it a useful tool to support the pupils to know when they should access a sensory strategy.'

The ultimate goal of using sensory strategies is that the pupil will be able to identify their own arousal level and choose an appropriate strategy to support themselves. At the beginning, all pupils need adult support to access sensory strategies. However, over time and with support they can become more independent.

Teaching tip

Emotional regulation programmes work best when they are implemented across the whole school. This means that all teachers are using the same language and will understand how to support the pupils who need the strategies the most.

There are a number of different programmes available to help pupils to identify their emotional states and which strategies they can use to help themselves to regulate. All of these use a combination of colours and/or numbers to identify different states of arousal. They start by teaching pupils what high and low arousal feels like. Then they help to plot an individual plan for the pupil that includes strategies to help them to calm down or become more alert.

Programmes include:

- Emotions Toolbox
- Sensory Ladders
- Zones of Regulation
- Incredible 5-Point Scale
- Feel It Change It.

Initially, pupils need to be taught when to use strategies and what strategies will help to support them. The long-term goal is that they are independent, but this takes time and teaching. Some pupils can self-monitor when they are slightly dysregulated; however, if they are in overload or meltdown, they will likely need adult support to choose the best strategy.

Handwashing

'It took a very long time for him to start washing his hands at school. It seemed that it was the feeling of the soap.'

Handwashing can be tricky for some pupils. Usually, these pupils experience some touch sensitivity, and the texture of the water, soap or towel is a challenge. Occasionally, there can be difficulty with the planning or scents.

Some things to try for pupils with touch sensitivity:

- If the pupil is verbal, you can ask what part of handwashing they find difficult, and adapt it.
- If the pupil is non-verbal, you can observe them during play with the different textures to see whether one is more difficult than another, e.g. do they engage in water play?
- Consider the scent of the soap, as sometimes this can be the issue.
- If running water is the issue, consider using the plug and making a small pool of water.
- Consider the type of soap. Bar soap can become very sticky when it is left wet. However, it is less sticky when dry. Pre-foaming soap is also a different texture to liquid soap. See what the pupil prefers.
- If the pupil likes the feeling of the 'therapressure' brush (Idea 45), check to see whether they would be comfortable using this to wash their hands.
- Think about the towel and try different towel textures.

Considering dyspraxia

Pupils with dyspraxia might need help when they need to use a new tap or soap dispenser. Double check that moving what to do when moving classrooms or in an unfamiliar environment. Sometimes, they might just need a demonstration.

Teaching tip

If there happens to be a hand dryer, this could be the reason why the pupil is avoiding washing their hands. In this case, it's likely they find the sound of the dryer overwhelming. So, give them an alternative and let them use the space without others turning the dryer on.

Material organisation in class

'He is forever losing things; even his PE kit has gone missing once already this term. There is just no organisation at all.'

Some pupils, particularly those with dyspraxia, struggle to keep their materials organised. They frequently lose items. As they get older, they don't arrive with the correct items for lessons. It often takes them longer to get ready for lessons as well.

Some strategies you can use to support these pupils include:

- See-through pencil cases and folders can help them to see where items are more easily.
- Pencil cases or bags with compartments for each item can help to make sure everything is packed away.
- Pupils could have their own tray or space to store items to which they are always directed.
- Colour-code books so that each subject has a different colour and is easily recognised.
- Write a list of items required for that subject on the front of its exercise book to refer to.
- Have a list at the front of the class of items the pupil needs to have ready on their desk.
- If the pupil struggles to keep items in their space, a coloured placemat for them to put items on can sometimes help.
- If they are really struggling, you can also mark stationery outlines onto the placemat to show them where to put their items when they aren't using them.
- Teach the pupil to have a 'proper look' for items around their desk when tidying away, including looking under their desk.
- Have a folder for any documents that need to go between home and school.
- A checklist of items for the school bag can help (e.g. homework or reading book).

Bonus idea ★

Pupils with dyspraxia may need explicit practice in getting ready for subjects. So, spend some time demonstrating and practising getting their books and stationery ready. This way, they know the routine for when they need to do it in lessons.

Difficulty in PE

'She always struggled in PE. Catching a ball was so hard for her. She just never seemed to be able to coordinate or time her movements.'

PE is typically a very hard subject for pupils with dyspraxia. In addition, it can be quite overwhelming for pupils with sensitivities due to the increased noise, touch and movement. Pupils with slower responses might find getting started and also balance activities harder.

When supporting pupils in PE, it is first important to understand their sensory patterns. These are explored in Part 2 of this book. Each pattern will have slightly different needs in PE.

Pupils with dyspraxia (Idea 10) will need more time to learn new activities. They will need extra demonstrations and time to practise. If you are teaching specific sports each term, e.g. football, it can help if their parents know this in advance so they can start to practise at home. Ideas 50 to 52 also give additional suggestions.

Pupils with sensory sensitivities can be easily overloaded during a PE lesson. Typically, PE is loud. There is usually movement and there are many opportunities for accidental touch, so the pupil is processing all of these additional sensations. They may need extra breaks during PE to regulate. It can also be helpful to bring items that support regulation (e.g. ear defenders) to the lesson to have them on hand.

Pupils who are slower to process sensory inputs are likely to take longer to get organised. Their performance will likely be better towards the middle of the lesson. Make sure to include jumping and running in their warm-up to help increase arousal. Be mindful that they may fatigue more quickly than others and may need a shorter lesson initially, though a long-term goal is to increase endurance.

Teaching tip

Pupils with sound sensitivity may find whistles a challenge. Consider the sound your whistle makes and how loudly you blow it. In some cases, bird call whistles with a softer pitch can be a helpful alternative.

Helping parents

Part 10

Home and school communication

'We have a simple exercise book in which we just note down any differences through the day. His parents let us know about sleep and any changes going on at home. It's really helpful to have the line of communication open.'

Home and school communication is absolutely essential for success. The pupil spends more than half of their time at home and this will impact their regulation. Equally, the events of the school day will impact arousal levels at home.

Teaching tip

Some pupils may feel more comfortable expressing their concerns at home, rather than in school. An open communication system will allow parents to easily feed this information back to the class teacher.

The school environment and policies will dictate the easiest way for this to occur. In some cases, verbal handovers can be done. In others, a book is required. Even with verbal handovers, it can be helpful to keep a record of the information, as this can help with pattern identification if there are challenges.

Useful information to know from home includes sleep, toileting routine (including constipation), changes to routine, e.g. visitors or a birthday party, triggers that have been noticed and what's working well. Helpful information to hand over from school includes what went well during the day, any strategies that helped, triggers, challenges that occurred in the day and anything out of the ordinary in the pupil's behaviour.

Bonus idea ★

If you're using a communication book, pictures, e.g. smiley, straight and sad faces or numbers, can help to give a quick indication of how the day was.

For new pupils, parent information is vital. Find out all you can about the pupil's sensory preferences, what triggers them and what strategies help them to regulate. Not all strategies will be transferrable to school, but you will have a starting point. For existing pupils, it's still important to keep communication channels open. Pupils' needs and preferences change as they develop, and changes at home will continue to impact at school and vice versa.

Differences at home and at school

'I just don't understand – we have no issues at school, but his parents are reporting significant meltdowns at home.'

It is common for pupils to have varied sensory differences at home and school. Firstly, this is because the environmental and task demands are different. Secondly, there are activities that only occur at home and are not seen at school, e.g. teeth and hair brushing.

It is important to recognise that some pupils will internalise their overload (Idea 32) at school and then externalise it at home. They may appear 'fine' at school, but actually they are not. They are *managing*, but then they have a meltdown once they arrive home. Schools must understand and acknowledge that this pattern occurs for some families. They should work with the pupil and their family to help to reduce the overload the pupil is experiencing across their school day. Regulation activities might need to be completed by families before coming to school. Differences in the pupil's presentation across settings can be a trigger for conflict between school and home. It is important that parents' concerns and feedback are listened to. Teachers and parents should work together to create a solution that will best support the pupil.

Some parents may also need support to put in place strategies and consistency at home. The pupil may be successful at school, as it is structured and predictable, but there is less predictability at home. Sharing strategies that are successful at school may help at home. A referral for additional occupational therapy support, or in some cases social care, may also be relevant.

> **Teaching tip**
>
> At school, sometimes small changes with timetabling, like starting five minutes later than other pupils, can reduce overload in the morning.

> **Bonus idea** ★
>
> Having a designated support staff member, or key attachment figure, can also help the pupil to become more comfortable in school.

Using sensory strategies at home

'Mum continued with the yoga at home and had also made a calm space under the bed in her bedroom.'

Sensory strategies are not just for school! All of the strategies in this book are relevant for use at home as well. Pupils may have different sensory needs at home, but the principles remain the same.

Teaching tip

It is also really useful if the same language is being used at home and school. So, if school is using an emotional regulation programme, it is useful to teach this to the family as well.

Home and school communication (Idea 91) can help to create open dialogue between home and school about which strategies work when. A strategy helping at school may be suitable for home and vice versa. Parents can also help to support sensory needs and regulation at home before and after school. With some strategies, there is much more flexibility about how they can be used at home. Parents can easily give their children a hug, but as they get older it is not appropriate for teachers to hug pupils. Parents can add in a massage after the bath or before bed to help to support regulation but this is not a strategy that can be used before a maths lesson!

Sensory diets and calm spaces will look different at home and school due to the different environment, space and equipment available, but are still relevant strategies for both spaces. Pupils may need two pieces of some equipment – one for home and one for school. Other equipment may only be relevant for home. It's also useful to remember that some pupils don't like to transfer strategies between settings. These pupils might need a completely different set of ideas for home and school as they will link the strategy to the environment. This can occur frequently in autism, as the pupil will associate a strategy with a place or a person.

Useful sports and extra-curricular activities

'He was swimming twice a week and this seemed to really help his endurance.'

Many pupils participate in extra-curricular activities. They can be a great way to make friends and improve self-esteem. Sports can help with regulation. They are also a fantastic way to help with coordination.

It is important to find an activity that the pupil enjoys, rather than participating because it *should* be helpful. Pupils with sensory sensitivity sometimes find it hard to manage an extra activity on school days, so weekends may be better. You could discuss the following options at parents' evening.

Sports that can help with regulation

- swimming
- cycling
- yoga
- rock-climbing
- hiking
- horse riding.

Sports to help coordination

- martial arts, e.g. judo or karate – find a local club rather than a specific martial art type
- swimming
- playball
- athletics
- gymnastics
- rock-climbing
- yoga.

Non-sporting options can also help with developing self-esteem, such as drama clubs, Scouts/Brownies, LEGO® clubs and game clubs (both online and offline).

> **Teaching tip**
>
> Some pupils benefit from initial one-to-one lessons to help them to gain confidence before joining a larger group, especially for swimming.

> **Bonus idea** ★
>
> For pupils who have a specific diagnosis, there are also para-football leagues and community playgroups or meet-ups that may be relevant. You will need to check what is available in the local area.

Hair brushing and cutting

'She just won't let me brush her hair in the morning. It's a frequent trigger for a meltdown.'

Difficulty with hair brushing and cutting is commonly reported by parents of pupils with sensory sensitivities. In particular, it's reported by those who have touch sensitivity. Haircuts can be very difficult to manage. Here are some tips you can share with parents if they need support.

Teaching tip

Once the individual is old enough, teaching them to brush their own hair can be really helpful.

Tips for hair brushing

- Experiment with different hair brushes. Some individuals like the plastic bristles of a Tangle Teezer®, whilst others prefer soft brushes.
- It can be helpful to do some whole-body heavy work (Idea 59) before brushing begins.
- Start with a quite firm massage or squash on the head to help decrease sensitivity.
- In some cases, it can help to keep one hand with firmer pressure on one side of the head whilst brushing the hair on other side; this is much easier to do with short hair.
- Often a firmer brushing style, rather than being really light, can be more successful.
- It can also sometimes be helpful to have a countdown timer or to sing a song that the pupil knows so they understand when the hair brushing will be finished.

Additional tips for hair cutting

- Cutting hair at home can be a real life-saver. There are mobile hairdressers, and many families actually do their own.
- At the salon, pick a time when it's quieter.
- Scissors can be more successful than clippers as the buzzing noise can be difficult for those who also have sound sensitivity
- Practise going to the hairdresser. Practise with toys going to the hairdresser and use social stories if appropriate.

Bonus idea ★

Some individuals also find it helpful to do some sucking or chewing whilst their hair is being brushed. This can be achieved by drinking through a straw or with chewing gum or a chew toy.

Nail cutting

'She just won't let me cut her nails; we usually do it when she is sleeping.'

Nail cutting can also be tricky for those with sensory sensitivities. A lot of parents will cut their child's nails in their sleep to avoid the distress. Toenails are usually as difficult as fingernails. Here is some advice you can give to parents.

General tips

* Clippers are typically easier to use than scissors as there is less fiddling to get them into place. The feel of the clipper base gives more deep touch pressure than the feel of scissors going under the nail.
* Nails are usually softer and easier to cut after a bath or shower.
* Have the pupil do some heavy work beforehand (Idea 59) as this helps to prepare.

Cutting

1. Before cutting, ask the pupil to squeeze their hands for a count of five, ten times, to increase the proprioceptive sensory input.
2. Before putting the clippers onto the pupil's fingernail, give the fingertip a squeeze first.
3. When cutting, it can also help to squeeze the part of the finger you're holding.

The firmer touch pressure activates the discriminative touch pathway. This pathway is more calming than the protective touch pathway, which is activated by light touch. If nail cutting can be done with added proprioceptive (Idea 59) and touch pressure (Idea 44) sensory inputs, this will help to keep the pupil regulated.

Teaching tip

Teach the pupil to cut their nails themselves as soon as they are able.

Bonus idea ★

For some individuals, offering to paint their nails after cutting them can also be a good motivator.

Tooth brushing

'It took nearly a year to get him to brush his teeth. We tried sticker charts and bribery, but in the end the silicone toothbrush was the solution.'

Tooth brushing can be a challenge for pupils with touch sensitivity. There are so many sensory touch receptors in the mouth that the feel of the toothbrush can be overwhelming. Sometimes, there is also a dislike of the strong taste of the toothpaste. The following are ideas you can share with parents in this situation.

Prepare first without the toothbrush

Initially, it can be helpful to increase the pupil's tolerance of having different textures in their mouth. Try with a mirror and long pieces of carrot or a bread stick. Have the pupil rub this along their teeth, right to the back, tap their teeth and make sounds and pretend that it is a toothbrush and make the tooth-brushing motions. Add in pretend play with toys brushing their teeth during playtime, or try using social stories.

Getting ready to brush

Try some heavy work (Idea 59) prior to tooth brushing, or biting down on a sensory chew (Idea 75) for a minute before brushing can add proprioceptive sensory feedback. The proprioceptive input received from the jaw muscles could help to regulate them.

Tips for brushing

Electronic toothbrushes can be easier than regular ones, though the noise won't work for all pupils. Experiment with bristle hardness and softness. Silicone finger brushes can be helpful as they are a different texture to bristles. Use a brushing app with a countdown timer (e.g. NHS BrushDJ) or a song to help with timing, and use flavour-free toothpaste.

Bonus idea ★

Videos of others brushing their teeth can also help to show the pupil the routine of brushing, especially if it's their favourite TV characters, or a favourite friend or relative. There are also tooth brushing songs on YouTube by some of the characters kids love, like Hey Duggee and Super Simple.

Clothing

'Socks and shoes are a big problem; we really struggled with her tie.'

Difficulty with clothing textures, seams and tags is commonly reported by those with touch sensitivity. This can range from a preference for specific materials to a preference for tighter clothes or in some cases looser clothes. Some pupils will only wear specific brands and will wear the same favourite pieces of clothing over and over.

If you have a pupil who struggles with clothing, it can help to have some flexibility with school uniforms, especially at the start. These pupils will likely find ties and buttoned collars much harder to manage than t-shirts. They will also likely struggle with certain materials.

There is a large range of sensitivity-friendly clothing available in stores nowadays, including larger retailers (e.g. M&S seam-free range or Asda's 'Easy On Easy Wear' range), so make sure parents are aware of where they can find these items locally. Usually, the fabrics are softer and there are fewer seams. Cutting the tags out is an easy solution if the tag is a problem for the pupil.

There are a number of different suppliers for socks. These are usually labelled as 'seam-free'. Nowadays, they come in a variety of colours. Softer shoes, e.g. trainers, can also be more successful than solid leather shoes.

Some pupils will prefer the feel of clothing after it has been washed a few times to make it softer. Some may find tighter clothing (Idea 72) helpful to wear as a base layer. Also, the strategies for touch sensitivity in Part 5 will likely be relevant to help with decreasing overall sensitivity.

> **Teaching tip**
>
> Touch sensitivity can increase at times of stress or illness. So, if a pupil suddenly finds their clothing more uncomfortable than normal, consider whether there are any stress triggers or illness.

Body awareness activities for home

'We made a giant mess with the sofa, but it was so much fun! He loved the sandwiching!'

Poor body awareness does not stop when the pupil leaves the school gate! If it can be supported at home alongside school, the pupil will have more opportunities for practice. You might like to suggest some of the following activities to parents.

Activities for the garden

- sandpits
- potting plants
- digging
- water play, including using a watering can
- hide and seek
- football.

Activities for inside the home

- sandwiching between cushions or beanbags
- hide and seek, including 'can you fit inside or under'-type games
- rolling up and rolling out of duvets or sleeping bags
- rolling in a straight line
- console games with movement controllers such as the Nintendo® Wii.

Activities for outside the home

- playground equipment
- climbing frames
- cycling
- swimming
- hiking
- martial arts.

Creating a sensory lifestyle

'It doesn't stop at the school gate, nor should it be scheduled in at a specific time. The best way to achieve success is to create a sensory lifestyle.'

The final recommendation in this book is to create a sensory lifestyle. By doing this, sensory strategies will become part and parcel of the pupil's day. They won't be another thing to 'fit in' and they won't be forgotten. The pupil's entire lifestyle will be supporting their regulation.

In order to achieve this, there needs to be successful collaboration between home and school. The pupil's sensory needs must be identified. Any patterns of behaviours should be noted, including times of or triggers for overload. Then, a plan can be made.

For example, if the pupil needs extra heavy work to regulate, can they cycle to school? Is there a climbing frame on the way to school or can they use the school one before lessons? What can be done through the school day to top this up? How can extra heavy work be added on the way home or at home?

If the pupil needs more downtime, where can this be scheduled as part of the normal routine? Can they join clubs with a later start time to add a gap between finishing school and starting something else? Can they do homework in the morning or have a break before starting it after school?

It is important to have a few quick supports that can be used at times of unexpected overload, or high or low arousal, but the aim is to embed supports into the daily routine, to become part of a lifestyle where the pupil's regulation and arousal are supported naturally throughout their day. It should be just something that happens naturally.

> **Teaching tip**
>
> It's also a great idea to include the pupil in the decision-making and planning. This means their ideas are being heard as well!

References

Ayres, A.J. (2005), *Sensory Integration and the Child: Understand Hidden Sensory Challenges* (25th anniversary edn). Los Angeles, CA: Western Psychology Services.

Ben-Sasson, A., Gal, E., Fluss, R. Katz-Zetler, N. and Cermak, S.A. (2019), 'Update of a meta-analysis of sensory symptoms in ASD: A new decade of research'. *Journal of Autism and Developmental Disorders*, 49, 4974–4996.

Crasta, J.E., Salzinger, E., Lin, M.-H., Gavin, W.J. and Davies, P.L. (2020), 'Sensory processing and attention profiles among children with sensory processing disorders and autism spectrum disorders'. *Frontiers in Integrative Neuroscience*, 14, 22.

Ghanizadeh, A. (2011), 'Sensory processing problems in children with ADHD, a systematic review'. *Psychiatry Investigation,* 8(2), 89–94.

Isaac, V., Olmedo, D., Aboitiz, F. and Delano, P.H. (2017), 'Altered cervical vestibular-evoked myogenic potential in children with attention deficit and hyperactivity disorder'. *Frontiers in Neurology*, 8, 90.

Kirby, A. and Cleaton, M. (2019), 'Neurodiversity 101: Co-occurrence'. Available online at: https://doitprofiler.com/wp-content/uploads/2019/07/ND101-What-is-co-occurrence-and-why-important.pdf

Parham, D., Cohn, E,. Spitzer, S., Koomar, J.A., Miller, L.J. Burke, J.P., Brett-Green, B., Mailloux, Z., May-Benson, T., Smith Roley, S., Schaaf, R.C., Schoen, S.A. and Summers, C.A. (2007), 'Fidelity in sensory integration intervention research'. *American Journal of Occupational Therapy*, 61, 216–227. Available online at: https://doi.org/10.5014/ajot.61.2.216

Further reading

Summary of links

Visit www.GriffinOT.com/100ideas for a full list of website links in the book, listed by idea number.

You can also join the free introductory sensory training to learn even more about the senses and sensory processing with Kim.

Introductory books on sensory processing

Allen, S. (2014), *Can I Tell You About Sensory Processing Difficulties?* London: Jessica Kingsley.

Dunn, W. (2009), *Living Sensationally.* London: Jessica Kingsley.

Miller, L. (2014), *Sensational Kids.* USA: Penguin Random House.

More in-depth books on sensory processing

Ayres, A. J. (2005), *Sensory Integration and the Child: Understand Hidden Sensory Challenges* (25th anniversary edn). Los Angeles, CA: Western Psychological Services.

Garland, T. (2014), *Self-Regulation Interventions and Strategies.* Eau Claire, Wisconsin: Pesi Publishing & Media.

Reebye, P. and Stalker, A. (2008), *Understanding Regulation Disorders of Sensory Processing in Children.* London: Jessica Kingsley.

Sensory processing and autism

Bogdashina, O. (2016), *Sensory Perceptual Issues in Autism and Asperger Syndrome* (2nd edn). London: Jessica Kingsley.

Grandin, T. (2006), *Thinking in Pictures.* London: Bloomsbury.

Higashida, N. (2014), *The Reason I Jump.* London: Sceptre.

Yack, E., Aquilla, P. and Sutton, S. (2015), *Building Bridges Through Sensory Integration* (3rd edn). Arlington, TX: Future Horizons.

Using sensory supports at school

Griffin, K. (forthcoming), *Success with Sensory Supports: The ultimate guide to using sensory diets, movement breaks, and sensory circuits at school.* London: Jessica Kingsley.

Explaining sensory processing to children

Brunker, L. (2014), *The Kids' Guide to Staying Awesome and In Control*. London: Jessica Kingsley.

Christmas, J. (2012), *Sensory Dinosaurs*. Oxford: Routledge.

Gianetti, M. and Russita, T. (2017), *Emily's Sister*. Lancaster: Your Stories Matter.

Books for parents

Introductory books above plus:

Kranowitz, C. (2005), *The Out-of-Sync Child*. New York, NY: Perigee.

Attachment/ADHD resources

Beacon House (2017), 'The repair of early trauma: A bottom up approach' [video]. YouTube. Available online at: www.youtube.com/watch?v=FOCTxcaNHeg

Lloyd, S. (2016), *Improving Sensory Processing in Traumatized Children*. London: Jessica Kingsley.

Maté, G. (2019), *Scattered Minds*. London: Vermilion.

Neufeld, G. and Maté, G. (2019), *Hold on to Your Kids*. London: Vermilion.

van der Kolk, B. (2015), *The Body Keeps the Score*. London: Penguin.

Meditation apps/resources

Headspace: www.headspace.com

Scope Mindful Monsters: https://mindfulmonsters.co.uk

Smiling Mind: www.smilingmind.com.au

Emotional regulation programmes

Feel It Change It: www.griffinot.com/feel-it-change-it

Emotions Toolbox: www.childtherapyservice.org.uk

Incredible 5-Point Scale: www.5pointscale.com

Sensory Ladders: https://sensoryladders.org

Zones of Regulation: www.zonesofregulation.com